Baby Care

C000017395

A handbook for mothers and health care students

Dr Winifred Kaine
MBBS, DCH, FRCP, FMCPaed.
Associate Professor and Consultant Paediatrician

The author and publishers would like to thank
   Professor O. Ransome-Kuti
      Director, Institute of Child Health,
      University of Lagos Teaching Hospital
and **Mrs A. Bailey**
      General Series Editor, Macmillan Tropical Nursing and
      Health Sciences Series
for their comments and advice on the manuscript.

This publication has been supported by a grant from
Cow and Gate Limited in the interests of public health education.

Ⓜ MACMILLAN

First published 1984
Reprinted 1985, 1986, 1988, 1992

Published by THE MACMILLAN PRESS LTD
London and Basingstoke
*Associated companies and representatives in Accra,
Auckland, Delhi, Dublin, Gaborone, Hamburg, Harare,
Hong Kong, Kuala Lumpur, Lagos, Manzini, Melbourne,
Mexico City, Nairobi, New York, Singapore, Tokyo.*

ISBN 0–333–36002–8

Printed in Hong Kong

Acknowledgements

The author and publishers wish to acknowledge, with thanks, the following photographic sources.

Church Missionary Society   p 88
Cow and Gate Limited   pp 6; 29; 69; 71 right; 98, 104; and the colour section
John and Penny Hubley   pp viii; 22; 78 top; 90
Institute of Child Health   pp 78 bottom; 126
Camilla Jessel   pp 76; 127
Mr M. O. Nwamoh   pp 5; 7; 16; 25
Rex Parry   pp 15; 33; 35; 66; 94; 96; 110
Popperfoto   p 41
UNICEF   p 24 photo by D. Anand
WHO   pp 13; 71 left photos by J. Mohr; 14; 20 photo by Eric Schwab; 78 bottom; 86 photos by M. Jacot; 121; 124
Zeal Limited   p 120 top
Cover photograph   Tony Stone Associates

The author and publishers also wish to thank the following for their help:
The Boots Company Limited for the loan of the baby foods, bottle brush, measuring jug, flask, pan and other equipment used in some of the photographs.
Mothercare for the loan of the baby clothing, weaning utensils, and other equipment used in some of the photographs.
Many thanks to Dr (Mrs) Felicia Jegede and her baby, Master Egwomaron Jegede, for sitting for the cover photograph.

The publishers have made every effort to trace the copyright holders but if they have inadvertently overlooked any, they will be pleased to make the necessary arrangements at the first opportunity.

Contents

Foreword

Dr Kaine is to be commended for writing what is, to our knowledge, the first general book on baby care written for mothers in Africa, with relevance to the Caribbean and other tropical areas.

This book is an expansion of a smaller booklet of notes for mothers, which Dr Kaine wrote and distributed on her own initiative, in response to the needs of mothers attending the hospital where she is now Head of the Department of Paediatrics. This much-needed volume includes all aspects of the health and care of babies from birth to twenty-four months, richly illustrated with diagrams and photographs.

Baby Care is aimed at those who can read, in English, up to and beyond secondary school level, and who are aware of the value of books on public health education. It is assumed that the facilities and equipment available to such readers will be fairly good and that the standards to which they aspire will be fairly high.

Health care students on a variety of courses, especially student midwives and nurses, and community health workers are recommended to use this book, in their studies and as reference, in their daily work.

The main beneficiaries of this book, however, will be our children who will grow up happy and healthy if their mothers and families follow the excellent and well-presented advice contained in it. Having been involved ourselves in promoting improved health care and in public health education, we are pleased to have been asked to advise on Dr Kaine's most welcome book, and we congratulate her on her efforts.

Professor O. Ransome-Kuti
Mrs A. Bailey

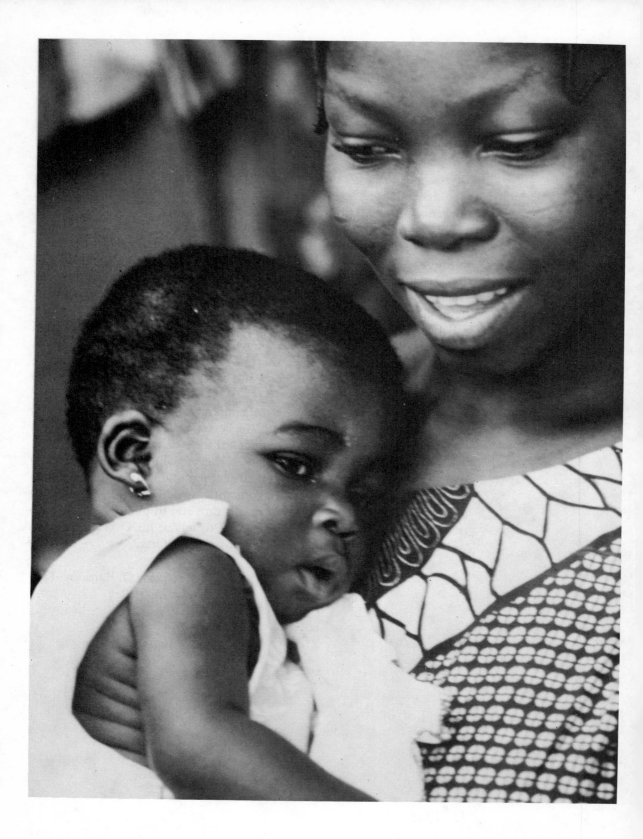

1   Pregnancy

Pregnancy is a natural process, not a disease. Our ancestors had the right attitude towards it; they went about their normal business during pregnancy and looked after themselves as well as they could. Unfortunately, many modern women regard it as a time of illness with the result that they develop unnecessary psychological problems when they are pregnant.

The life of a baby begins from the moment it is conceived. At birth, the baby is actually nine months or forty weeks old. The purpose of pregnancy is to provide the unborn baby with the ideal conditions in which to develop from a simple egg into a complicated human being. An unborn baby is known as a **foetus**[1].

The stages of pregnancy

Pregnancy is divided into three stages, each lasting three months. Each stage is known as a **trimester**. The first, second and third trimesters each refer to the first, second and final three months of pregnancy, respectively. These stages are summarised on page 2.

First trimester

The first trimester is the most crucial period in the life of the foetus. During this period, the foetus develops from an egg into a recognisable human being by means of a delicate and complicated process. If anything goes wrong, it may lead to foetal death, followed by abortion, or to severe deformity of the foetus. It is a well-known fact that most miscarriages occur during the first three months of pregnancy. It is not so well known that babies born with deformities may well have suffered damage during early pregnancy. For example, expectant mothers who get German measles, or rubella, at this stage could cause damage to their baby. Expectant mothers should also be very careful about the drugs they take at this stage. The case of the **thalidomide** drug is an example of the harmful effects caused by some drugs.

The womb undergoes considerable changes during the first trimester. These changes result in the formation of the **placenta**. This is the vehicle through which the foetus receives its nourishment and through which it disposes of its waste products. It is joined to the foetus by the **umbilical cord**. By the end of the first trimester, the womb has more than trebled in size and can be felt at the lower end of the expectant mother's abdomen.

1. All words in bold type are explained in the Glossary on page 131.

1

The stages of pregnancy

First trimester

The foetus develops in the shelter of the womb. This is a delicate process and many deformities can occur at this stage. There is a risk of miscarriage throughout this stage of pregnancy.

The placenta forms to provide nourishment through the umbilical cord.

The fluid surrounding the foetus provides protection.

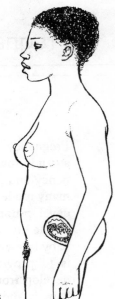

at 12 weeks

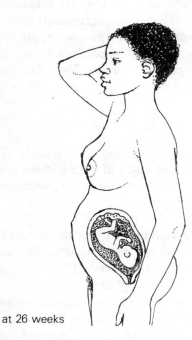

Second trimester

This stage is more stable and there is far less risk of miscarriage.

The foetal organs become more mature and increase in size.

It is often possible to feel the various parts of the baby's body towards the end of this stage.

at 26 weeks

Third trimester

The foetus increases in size rapidly but must be given adequate nourishment to do so. The baby is usually born towards the end of the ninth month, after it has moved down towards the mother's birth canal in preparation for labour. However, babies born as early as the end of the seventh month can survive if cared for properly.

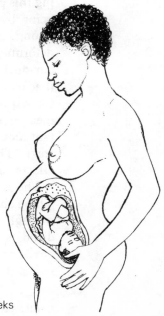

at 40 weeks

Second trimester

Pregnancy is more stable during the second trimester. The various foetal organs, which are developed during the first trimester, become more mature. The process of maturity is accompanied by an increase in size of the individual organs. By the end of the sixth month of pregnancy it is often possible to feel the head, trunk and limbs of the foetus. The womb has also increased in size, reaching to the level of the expectant mother's navel.

Third trimester

The third trimester is characterised by a rapid increase in the size of the foetus. This is due to rapid growth of the foetal bones and muscles and to the development of fatty tissue in various parts of the foetus. If the foetus does not get enough nourishment, the newborn baby will have a low birth weight. Such a baby is liable to develop serious problems. The rapid increase in size is accompanied by further maturity of the various organs. If a baby were born at the end of the seventh month of pregnancy, he[2] would then have a chance of survival if properly taken care of.

The end of the third trimester marks the end of pregnancy. If all has gone well, the foetus is then fully developed and ready to be born. The womb has by then reached to the top of the abdomen. However, its level may fall slightly in the last week or two as the baby's head drops towards the mother's birth canal in preparation for labour (see Fig 1.1).

2. The baby is referred to as 'he' throughout the book for the sake of clarity and simplicity.

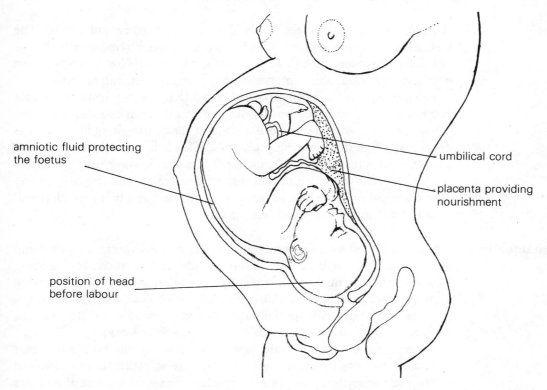

amniotic fluid protecting the foetus

umbilical cord

placenta providing nourishment

position of head before labour

Fig 1.1   Position of foetus towards the end of the third trimester.

Requirements of the foetus

Like all human beings, the foetus requires nourishment, shelter and protection against injury and disease.

Nourishment

This is provided by the mother through the blood she supplies to the placenta. She must therefore eat for herself as well as for the foetus. Nature tries to help by giving her a large appetite but she must take care that she does not put on too much weight.

Shelter

The womb provides an ideal shelter for the foetus. The **amniotic fluid** which surrounds the foetus acts as a shock absorber and helps to protect it against external injury.

Protection

Disease can only reach the foetus through its mother. If the mother is in good health and free from disease then the foetus is safe. The expectant mother's health is taken care of at the **antenatal clinic**.

Requirements of the expectant mother

The main requirements are good diet, regular check-ups at the antenatal clinic and routinely prescribed drugs.

Good diet

A good diet is essential for the health of both mother and foetus. The foetus is a complete parasite and will take whatever it requires whether or not the mother has enough left for her own needs. This is why women who have babies at short intervals are frequently thin and anaemic.

The diet in developing countries often contains too much starch and not enough protein. In other words, the people eat too much cassava, yam, maize, plantain and so on and not enough meat, fish or eggs. Protein is particularly important during pregnancy. This is because the foetus needs a lot of protein for growth. The mother's diet should also contain plenty of fruit and vegetables which provide essential vitamins, and also help to prevent constipation. Later on in this book, nutrition and balanced diets will be discussed in greater detail (see Chapter 7).

The antenatal clinic

The clinic is designed for the exclusive care of the expectant mother and her unborn baby. It is run by qualified midwives. A **midwife** is a nurse who, after her training in general nursing, undergoes specialised training in midwifery. This is a branch of medicine which deals with all aspects of pregnancy. In hospitals, specially trained doctors are also in attendance at antenatal clinics to deal with difficult or complicated cases.

All expectant mothers should register at an antenatal clinic when their pregnancy reaches a certain stage but the stage at which they are allowed to register varies from one clinic to another. Some clinics accept mothers as early as three months and others as late as five months after the begin-

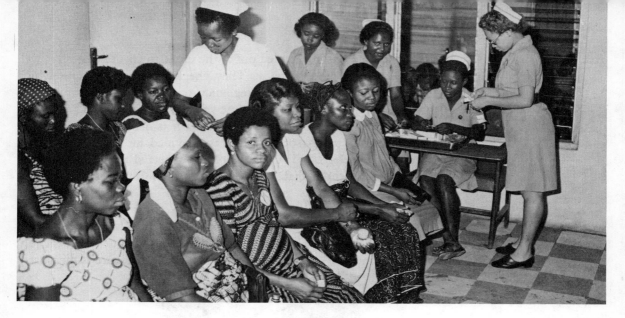

Fig 1.2   At the antenatal clinic.

ning of pregnancy. As soon as your pregnancy is confirmed, you should choose your antenatal clinic and register at the stage recommended by the clinic.

Registration

This is essentially the same as registration at other types of clinic. Your personal particulars are written on to a special **antenatal record card** by a records clerk. Your antenatal number is also written on a small **appointment card** which you keep with you and produce whenever you attend the clinic. The records clerk can easily find your antenatal card from the number on your appointment card. An antenatal card and an appointment card are shown in Fig 1.3 and Fig 1.4.

Fig 1.3   An antenatal card.

Fig 1.4   An antenatal appointment card.

PRIMARY ASSESSMENT	Date: / /

History of present pregnancy

BLEEDING	
DISCHARGE	
URINARY SYMPTOMS	D E T A I L S
SWELLING OF ANKLES	
OTHER SYMPTOMS	

Physical examination

		HEIGHT
GENERAL CONDITION	OEDEMA	WEIGHT
	ANAEMIA	B.P.
RESPIRATORY SYSTEM		URINE
CARDIOVASCULAR SYSTEM		BREAST & NIPPLES
ABDOMEN	SPLEEN CM	Hb.
	LIVER	GENOTYPE
		KAHN
VAGINAL EXAMINATION		GROUP, RH
		CHEST X-RAY
OTHER ABDOMALITIES		

EXAMINER:

normally completed by consultant at second visit

Comments

SIGNATURE:

Special instructions regarding puerperium

UNIVERSITY OF NIGERIA TEACHING HOSPITAL

Surname .... A.N.C. No ....

Other Names .... Age .... Date ....

Address ....

... .Blood Group ....

APPOINTMENT CARD	ANTENATAL DEPARTMENT

CONSULTANT:			Casenote No.		
Day	Next Date Visit	Time	Day	Next Date Visit	Time

Various examinations are carried out at the clinic to ensure that all is well with you and your unborn baby. They check for any conditions which might cause risk either during pregnancy or at delivery. Examinations (a) to (d) below are carried out each time you attend the clinic. The last two are carried out once and repeated only when it is necessary to do so.

a) *Urine examination.* A special room is provided for this examination. Fresh urine is preferred. You are therefore expected to produce a fresh specimen which is immediately tested for any abnormalities by a nurse.

b) *Blood pressure.* This is measured with a machine called a **sphygmomanometer**, shown in Fig 1.5. The strip of material or cuff is wrapped round your upper arm and inflated. This may cause some discomfort but no pain. The doctor or nurse listens to your heartbeat and, at the same time, the cuff is deflated as your blood pressure is measured.

Fig 1.5
A sphygmomanometer
in use.

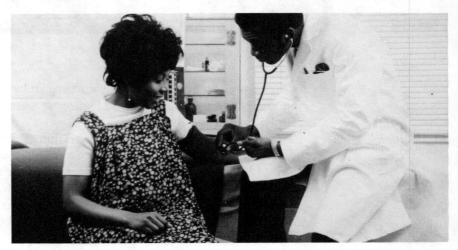

c) *Weight.* This is measured in order to ensure that you are gaining weight at the correct rate as your pregnancy advances. If you gain weight too slowly or too rapidly, it may mean that something has gone wrong.

d) *Abdominal examination.* This is known as a **palpation**. During the palpation, the size of the womb is assessed. The state of the foetus and its position are also determined. The midwife also listens to the foetal heartbeat, as shown in Fig 1.7. It is particularly important to know the position of the foetus as it may be necessary to correct it before it is too late. If the baby is not lying correctly before labour begins, it may require an operation known as a **Caesarian section** to bring the baby out.

e) *Vaginal examination.* This is done at your first visit to the antenatal clinic. The purpose of the examination is to find out if there is anything wrong so that it can be treated in time. In expectant mothers who are pregnant for the first time, the size of the pelvis is also assessed. This is to ensure that the baby has enough room to pass through during delivery. A few women have a small pelvis and can only have their babies by Caesarian section.

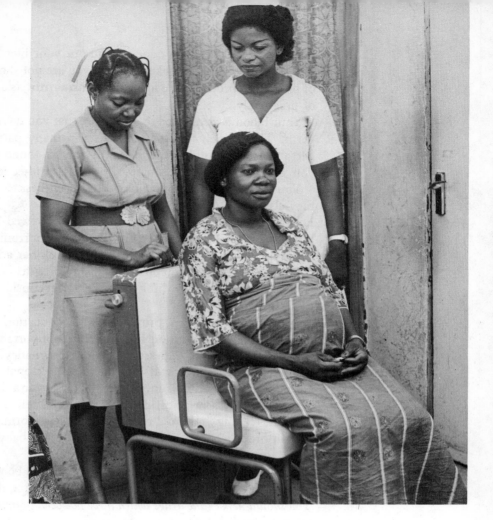

Fig 1.6
An expectant mother
being weighed at the
clinic.

Fig 1.7
Abdominal examination
of an expectant mother

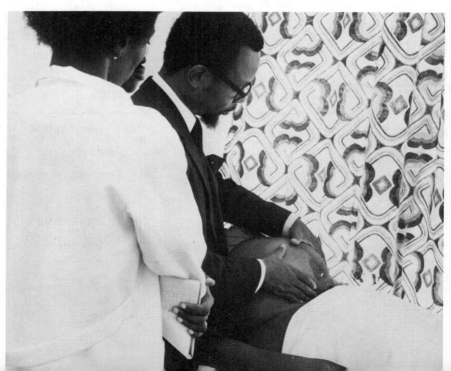

f) *Blood tests*. These are done to find out your blood group if this is not already known, and to make sure that you are not short of blood. Shortage of blood, the proper name for which is **anaemia**, is a serious complication of pregnancy.

Your blood is also tested to make sure that you do not carry the **syphilis** germ. This ancient disease still exists in many parts of the world. The germ is very harmful to the foetus. If you are found to harbour the germ, you will be placed on a course of **penicillin** injections.

You may be sent for other blood tests if necessary. Other examinations may also be done as the need arises.

Interview with the midwife

During your examination, you will be interviewed by the midwife. The purpose of the interview is to give you the opportunity to tell the midwife about any problems you may have or to seek her advice.

It is important that you do not keep anything from the midwife, no matter how trivial you may think it is. What you consider to be trivial may be quite important.

Health education

Some antenatal clinics provide health education for their expectant mothers. Health education is particularly important in countries where there is still a lot of superstition about pregnancy. It should consist of simple lectures and discussions on diet, personal hygiene and general cleanliness. Harmful superstitious beliefs and practices should be discouraged by a practical demonstration of their harmful effects.

Infant-feeding and child-rearing should also form part of health education in order to prepare the mother before her baby arrives.

Drugs

It should be stressed once more that you should be very careful about the drugs you take, particularly during the first three months of pregnancy. *You should never take drugs which have not been prescribed by a qualified doctor or midwife.*

The drugs which are routinely prescribed for expectant mothers in African countries are listed in Fig 1.8. Other drugs may be prescribed if necessary.

Drug	Form	Purpose
Iron	Tablet	To keep up blood levels and prevent anaemia
Folic acid	Tablet	As above
Multivite	Tablet	To maintain general health
Calcium	Tablet	To aid the development of foetal bones
Daraprim	Tablet	To prevent malaria
Tetanus toxoid	Injection	To prevent tetanus in the newborn baby

Fig 1.8 Drugs prescribed for expectant mothers.

Care of the nipple

A good nipple is essential for successful breast-feeding. If you have a flat or retracted nipple (see Fig 1.9) it should be treated during pregnancy. This is done by pulling on the nipple and massaging it between the fingers as often as possible whenever you undress and during your bath. Severe retraction of the nipple may require the wearing of a gadget known as a nipple-shield. This works by exerting constant pressure on the nipple, forcing it out of its retracted position. However, nipple-shields are very rarely used in African countries.

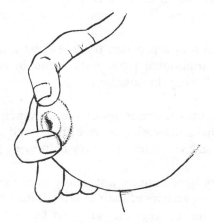

Fig 1.9   Massaging a retracted nipple.

Common problems

Many women go through pregnancy with few or no problems. A woman's attitude towards pregnancy has a profound effect on how she fares during pregnancy. Doctors are of the opinion that many of the problems of pregnancy are psychological in origin. It is essential to point out that although some problems are recognised as being complications of pregnancy, this does not mean that all expectant mothers will suffer from all of them. Some of the most common problems are discussed here.

Vomiting

Some women vomit during early pregnancy, mainly in the morning. Many others do not vomit at all. Some vomit only after they have been told that they are pregnant. Vomiting is sometimes accompanied by nausea. To overcome the feeling of sickness, you should try to eat very simple, dry food frequently.

Dizziness

This occurs in some women, mainly during early pregnancy. If dizziness occurs the expectant mother should not get up suddenly. It generally passes fairly quickly and does not require any special treatment. Anaemia, as the cause of dizziness, can be detected by means of a blood test.

9

Aches and pains	During the first trimester of pregnancy, there may be mild backache or waist pain. The pain may move to the abdomen in the second and third trimesters. In late pregnancy, the pressure of the womb on the lower part of the rib-cage may cause some discomfort in that area. Heartburn may occur, caused either by the pressure of the womb on the stomach or by the laxity of the opening at the upper end of the stomach. When the baby's head descends into the pelvis towards the end of pregnancy, backache may reappear or become more troublesome.
Craving for unusual foods	An increased appetite is normal during pregnancy and, in some expectant mothers, is accompanied by a craving for unusual foods. This craving is quite harmless provided that nothing poisonous is eaten!
A sour taste in the mouth	This is sometimes a problem for a few expectant mothers. Fortunately, some of the traditional bitter nuts found in African countries are very helpful in relieving the sourness.
Constipation	Pregnancy causes the muscles of the abdomen to relax. This relaxation sometimes make defecation more difficult and is liable to cause constipation. Fruits and vegetables are very helpful in preventing constipation.
Pimples and boils	Many women have pimples just before their menstrual periods as a result of the increased activity of their ovaries. These pimples may become more pronounced during pregnancy and may be complicated by boils. Washing frequently, preferably with a mild antiseptic soap, helps to reduce the number of pimples and to prevent boils.
Frequent urination	This is a normal feature of pregnancy. It is caused partly by the increased activity of various organs of the body and partly by the presence of an enlarged womb which reduces the space available for the bladder. This is the muscular sac where urine is stored before it is passed.
Itching of the genital organs	Itching may occur during pregnancy and may involve any part of the body, but is usually more noticeable in the genital organs, or private parts. It is probably caused by the various changes induced by pregnancy. Provided there is no rash or excessive vaginal discharge, it should not cause any alarm.
Vaginal discharge	Some women have a mild vaginal discharge just before their menstrual periods and when they are pregnant. It is caused by the increased activity of their ovaries. It is not offensive and does not cause itching. Copious vaginal discharge, especially if accompanied by an offensive odour or itching, is the result of an infection which requires treatment.
Swelling of the feet	Swelling of the feet usually appears during the second or third trimester in those who are prone to this complaint. It is the result of the pressure of the

pregnant womb on the blood vessels in the pelvis. It can be prevented or reduced by avoiding prolonged standing and by sitting with the legs raised. However, in some cases, swelling of the feet is an early sign of **toxaemia of pregnancy** so, if her feet do swell, the expectant mother should tell the midwife or doctor.

Piles and varicose veins

Piles or haemorrhoids are prominent, branching blood vessels situated in the anus. They show themselves by causing bleeding from the anus whenever the patient goes to the toilet. Varicose veins are large, prominent blood vessels which can be seen on the legs. Both piles and varicose veins are caused by pressure of the large womb on the blood vessels in the pelvis. Avoiding constipation helps to reduce bleeding from piles. Standing for prolonged periods is bad for varicose veins and should be avoided. Elastic bandages or stockings may help to reduce varicose veins. Fortunately, both piles and varicose veins usually disappear after pregnancy.

Bloating

The increased activity of the ovaries is responsible for the gain in weight and the bloated feeling which many women experience just before, as well as during, their menstrual period. The gain in weight results from the retention of too much salt and water in the body. The same process occurs during pregnancy and can be very pronounced in some expectant mothers. In some cases, bloating may be a sign of toxaemia of pregnancy.

Bleeding

There are two types of bleeding during pregnancy. One type produces small blood stains on the pants. It is known as 'spotting' and occurs during early pregnancy. It is caused by the changes taking place in the womb and is usually harmless. The second type produces more copious bleeding and is dangerous. It can occur at all stages of pregnancy and should be reported at once to the doctor or midwife.

Toxaemia of pregnancy

This is the most serious complication of pregnancy. However, the cause is still not clear. The disease shows itself by a swelling of the feet, a rise in blood pressure and the appearance of protein in the urine. It must be promptly treated, preferably in hospital.

What to avoid

Excessive eating

Too much of a good thing is bad. Excessive eating, especially of starchy food, leads to obesity. Obesity places extra strain on the heart, bones and joints and makes people more liable to develop diabetes and high blood pressure. It also reduces the efficiency of the muscles and other body organs. Finally, it may cause the foetus to become too large. Some of our more wealthy women eat far too much during pregnancy.

Smoking

Modern medicine has proved that excessive smoking during pregnancy affects the placenta and leads to the birth of a small baby. Low birth weight babies, as such babies are known, are liable to develop all sorts of complications. Smoking is not yet common amongst women in Africa but it may become a problem in the future.

Alcohol

Drinking alcohol in moderate quantities is not harmful. Excessive drinking is bad, whether one is pregnant or not. It has a bad effect on the foetus and may cause a dangerous condition known as **foetal-alcohol syndrome**. As with smoking, excessive drinking is not yet common amongst our women.

Sexual intercourse

Sexual intercourse should be avoided by expectant mothers whose pregnancy has threatened to abort, or who have aborted in the past. Other women may have sexual intercourse if they wish. However, some doctors feel that it is advisable to avoid intercourse during the first and last weeks of pregnancy in order to give the expectant mother maximum physical and emotional rest.

Heavy work

Many women can perform heavy physical work during pregnancy. However, other women cannot do so without endangering their pregnancy. Women who have had abortions in the past should avoid heavy work when they are pregnant.

Incorrect superstitions

Pregnancy is still associated with many superstitious beliefs which are incorrect and should not be taken seriously. The following are some of them.
1. Sitting near the fire in the first three months of pregnancy causes the foetus to melt.
2. Eating eggs, meat or fish during pregnancy results in the birth of a greedy child who likes to steal.
3. Eating snails makes the baby dribble saliva constantly after birth.
4. Drinking a lot of water causes excessive growth of the foetus.
5. Looking at ugly people, animals or objects results in the birth of a hideous baby.
6. Certain types of bush meat prolong labour whereas other types shorten it.

2 Birth

The best place to have a baby is in a hospital or a well-equipped maternity home. These institutions have the right facilities for a safe confinement and employ adequately trained personnel. It must be mentioned, however, that some maternity homes are poorly equipped and are run by poorly trained midwives. You should be careful to choose a good maternity home if you do not wish to have the baby in a hospital. It is advisable to have your baby where you had your antenatal care. This is because the staff are used to you and can easily recognise any new development in your case.

Ideally, expectant mothers who are pregnant for the first time, or who have had more than five children, should be delivered in a hospital. This is because labour complications tend to occur more frequently in these mothers, and are much better handled in a hospital.

In some tropical countries it may not be advisable for expectant mothers to have their babies at home because of the unhygienic conditions in some homes. Home confinement is still common in some areas and is usually supervised by traditional midwives, who have little or no idea of modern medical practice. Lack of proper antenatal care and inadequate home confinement facilities are largely responsible for the continuing high rate of maternal and infant deaths.

Fig 2.1   At a maternity home.

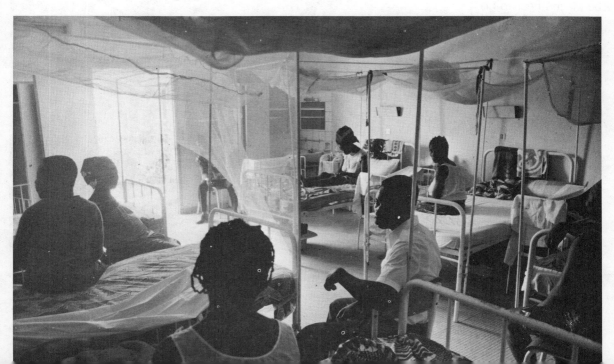

Preparing for the new baby

Many antenatal clinics provide expectant mothers with a list of items to be bought in preparation for the new baby. For the benefit of those who are not given such a list, the following are the main items:

a) a large bowl to act as a bath tub;

b) a soft face towel for bathing the baby and a large towel for drying his body;

c) mild baby soap for bathing and talcum powder for the nappy area;

d) olive oil for the baby's skin (not essential);

e) a small comb for the hair;

f) sterile dressings and bandages for the umbilical cord;

g) methylated spirit or gentian violet paint for the raw umbilicus;

h) good quality baby nappies with proper safety pins;

i) babies' waterproof pants;

j) cotton vests and gowns for warm weather, flannel vests and gowns for cool weather;

k) a kettle for boiling the baby's water and

l) a large flask in which to keep boiled water.

The room where the baby is to sleep should have plenty of light and air and should not be cluttered with household goods. If the parents can afford it, the baby should also have a separate cot placed close to his mother's bed (see Fig 2.2). The purpose of this semi-isolation of the new baby is to prevent cross-infection from the other members of the family. The purpose of a separate cot for the baby is to make it less easy for any infections, such as catarrh or a cough, to pass from the mother to the baby.

Fig 2.2
The baby's cot should be placed near to his mother's bed.

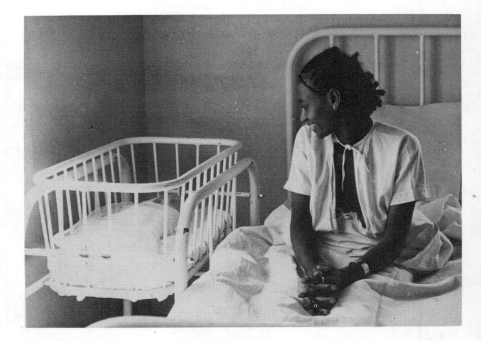

Labour

The first sign that labour has started is the discharge from the vagina of a small amount of slimy substance, or mucus, mixed with blood. It is caused by the separation of the membranes which line the womb from the neck of the womb. Labour ends with the delivery of the placenta or **afterbirth**. The duration of labour varies from one woman to another. As a rule, it is longest with the first pregnancy.

Stages of labour

Labour is divided into three stages. The first stage is the longest. The main event during the first stage is the gradual widening or dilation of the opening at the neck of the womb. This stage ends when the opening into the womb is fully dilated and forms a common channel with the vagina. The membranes rupture towards the end of this stage with the release of some of the fluid which surrounds the baby.

The second stage begins when the opening into the womb is fully dilated and ends with the birth of the baby. The strong desire to push, which many mothers experience at the beginning of this stage, is caused by the pressure of the baby's head on the floor of the vagina. The baby is born by the combined force of the powerful contractions of the womb and the downward push of the mother. It is important to follow the instructions of the midwife in order to avoid injury to the baby or to the vagina.

The third and final stage of labour begins after the birth of the baby. There is usually a short pause before the labour pains appear once more. This is nature's way of giving the mother a short rest after the rigours of the second stage. The third stage is the shortest. It ends with the birth of

Fig 2.3
Baby immediately after birth.

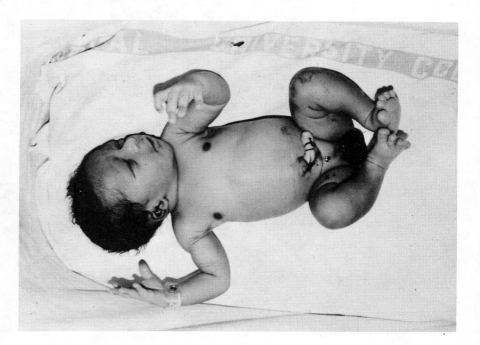

15

the placenta, called the afterbirth. An injection is sometimes given to the mother to make the third stage even shorter and also to prevent excessive bleeding.

Immediate care of the newborn baby

Immediately after birth, the baby is wrapped in a clean towel and taken to a cot where he is placed with his head slightly lower than his feet to encourage secretions to flow out. The mouth and nostrils are sucked clear of all liquid. The eyes are wiped clean with a sterile dressing. The baby is then carefully wrapped up and left to rest and recover from his recent experience. The old practice of instilling silver nitrate solution into the eyes is no longer recommended because it often causes inflammation of the baby's eyes. It is advisable to give the baby an injection of vitamin K to prevent an uncommon but dangerous bleeding disorder known as the haemorrhagic disease of the newborn. The injection may be given at this point or be delayed until after the baby's bath.

As soon as labour has ended and the mother has been made comfortable, the baby is given to her. This first contact between the mother and her baby is extremely important. It is the first step towards establishing a close bond between the two. **Bonding**, as the process is called, is essential for the normal development of the baby, as we shall see later.

Fig 2.4
Mother and newborn baby.

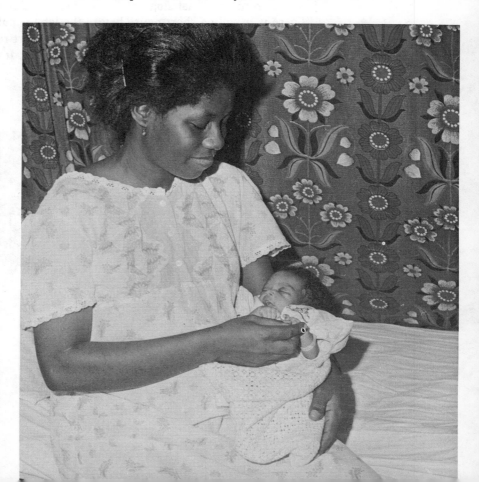

16

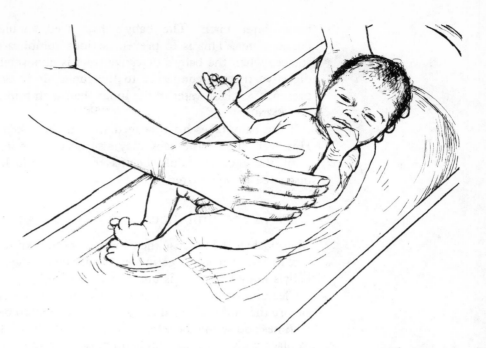

Fig 2.5
The baby's first bath.

Bathing

There are no hard and fast rules about when to give the newborn baby his first bath. The important thing is to remember that the baby needs a little time to recover from the rigours of being born. A waiting period of between half an hour and an hour will not do the baby any harm.

At birth, the newborn baby is covered with a protective creamy substance. The items required for the baby's first bath are warm water, soft soap and a face towel. After his bath, the baby may be rubbed gently all over with olive oil although this is not essential.

Clothing

The baby had no clothes on while he was in the womb. This enabled him to move freely within the confines of the womb. The newborn baby's clothing should be designed in such a way as to allow free movement. Tight clothing which may restrict movement or breathing is particularly dangerous.

Light, loose clothing is best for the newborn baby. Cotton clothing should be used in warm weather and flannel clothing in cool weather. Apart from a nappy and pants, a vest and a long gown are sufficient. The gown should have long sleeves and should reach well below the baby's feet. In a warm climate, there is usually no need for the woollen jumpers and socks in which some mothers are so fond of dressing their babies.

The first feed

Newly born babies are often seen placidly sucking their fists shortly after birth. This should not be mistaken for a sign of hunger. Most babies usually settle down for a long sleep soon after their first bath.

Again, there are no hard and fast rules about when to give the baby his first feed. Most babies are usually ready for a feed between six and twelve hours after birth. The baby's first feed should consist of a little boiled water. This is to prevent serious complications in those rare instances when the baby's digestive tract is abnormal, especially when the digestive tract is connected to the lungs. It is easier to deal with the presence of plain water in the lungs than with milk, no matter how small the quantity.

If the baby takes his first feed well, he can then be put to the breast. However, at first the baby may also need to be fed with glucose drinks until the mother's milk begins to flow well. Infant-feeding will be discussed in detail later.

Care of the umbilicus

Many babies die because their mothers do not know how to look after the umbilicus. Dangerous germs, especially tetanus germs, can enter into the baby's body through his umbilicus.

Cleanliness is the most important rule in the care of the umbilicus. Before the umbilical cord falls off, the area should be kept clean and dry at all times and should be covered with a sterile dressing. This should be kept in place with a bandage applied lightly around the baby's abdomen. Care must be taken to ensure that the bandage does not restrict breathing.

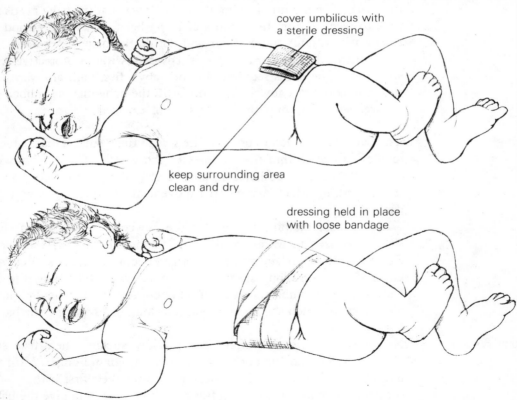

cover umbilicus with a sterile dressing

keep surrounding area clean and dry

dressing held in place with loose bandage

Fig 2.6   Correct bandaging of the umbilicus.

18

Plaster dressings should not be used as the newborn baby's delicate skin may be sensitive to the plaster. An antiseptic powder, prepared especially for the umbilical cord, can sometimes be obtained from the midwife before leaving the hospital or maternity home.

The umbilical cord should shrivel and fall off when the baby is between three and five days old. The raw umbilicus should be kept clean and dry as before and can, in addition, be painted with methylated spirit or gentian violet after cleansing. *However care must be taken here as methylated spirit can cause burns.* The umbilicus can then be left exposed, provided there is no infection. The practice of applying traditional medicine to the raw umbilicus is bad as the medicine invariably contains germs and other septic materials. With proper care, the umbilicus should be completely healed before the baby is ten days old.

Circumcision

In Africa, as in many parts of the world, the male newborn baby is often circumcised when he is seven or eight days old. The practice of circumcision is encouraged largely by culture and tradition. Many races do not practise circumcision and they do not suffer because of it.

The operation should be performed by a doctor or an experienced midwife, otherwise the baby may develop unnecessary complications. These take the form of bleeding or infection. The latter often leads to scarring and a narrowing of the hole in the baby's penis. This causes difficulties as it is then virtually impossible to get the hole back to its normal size.

Absolute cleanliness is essential in the care of the circumcision wound. Each time the baby soils himself, the penis should be gently, but thoroughly, cleaned after which an antiseptic cream or ointment should be applied. The baby may not be able to tolerate a nappy during the first few days after circumcision. In such cases, the nappy could be wrapped loosely around the baby's buttocks without touching the penis.

Different communities have their own traditional medicines for treating circumcision wounds. However, as in the case of the traditional umbilical medications, they often contain harmful germs, especially tetanus germs. Babies who develop **neonatal tetanus**, as the disease is called, do so through infection of the umbilicus or the circumcision wound. Such babies rarely recover.

Female circumcision

This practice still takes place in some parts of Africa in the mistaken belief that it promotes chastity. The operation is performed by an elderly man or woman in the village. Excessive bleeding and infection are the outcome in many cases. Infection leads to scarring and deformity of the female baby's genital organs with the result that the woman cannot give birth normally when she is an adult.

The first week of life

The first week is the most crucial in the life of all infants. It is known as the **perinatal period**. The newborn baby makes many important adjustments during this period. These adjustments are designed to help the baby exist successfully outside the womb. This is why circumcision is delayed until the end of the perinatal period.

The proportion of babies who are stillborn, or who die in the first week of life, is known as the **perinatal mortality**. It is a very accurate yardstick by which the stage of development of any nation can be measured. The perinatal mortality is still too high in Africa because of inadequate medical facilities.

Ideally, the newborn baby and his mother should not be discharged from the hospital or maternity home until after the perinatal period. This is so that the baby can be promptly taken care of should there be any problems. Unfortunately, because of lack of space, mothers and their babies are often sent home within twenty-four hours of confinement. Mothers are therefore advised to take their babies to the nearest hospital as soon as they suspect that something is wrong. Disorders which may occur include jaundice, tetanus and problems with breathing or feeding.

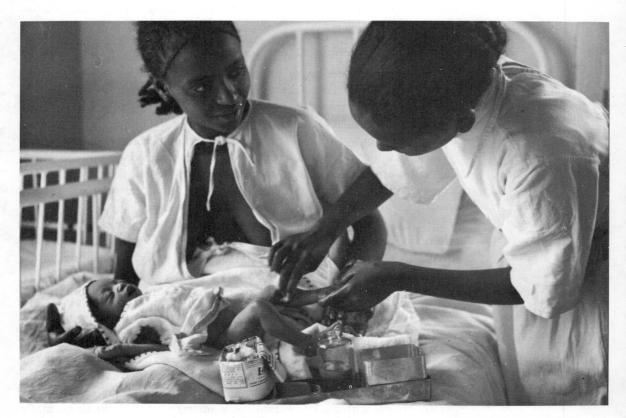

Fig 2.7   The mother and baby are well cared for by the medical staff.

3   Breast-feeding

Breast milk production

Breast milk is produced by glands which are present in the breasts of a female adult. These glands are not present in girls before adolescence, or in men. They are developed during adolescence or puberty. Their development is controlled by hormones which come from a gland at the base of the brain, stimulating the ovaries which, in turn, stimulate the development of the glands in the breast. It is not this process, however, which causes the secretion of the milk in the breast.

The secretion of milk by the fully developed breast is a separate process which is controlled directly by the brain. It starts during the second trimester of pregnancy and is one of the signs of advanced pregnancy. The secreted milk is stored inside the breast in readiness for the newborn baby. Its presence can be demonstrated by squeezing the breast.

The flow of milk is another process which is controlled by a special activity of the brain. The birth of the baby is the signal which sets the process in motion, but it may take two to three days before the flow of milk is fully established. It is important to note that *the amount of breast milk produced by an individual breast does not depend on the size of the breast*. Small breasts can produce quite large amounts of milk.

Conditions influencing milk production

Good diet

Your breast milk is made from ingredients in your blood. These ingredients are obtained from the food you eat. If your diet is well-balanced, there will be no shortage of ingredients, and your breasts will produce as much milk as is necessary. If your diet is inadequate, the ingredients will be obtained from your tissue and you will begin to lose weight. If you are badly underfed, this will reduce the amount of milk you produce. There is some evidence that in severe cases of malnutrition, the quality of the milk, as well as the quantity, may be altered but there is still no harm in trying to breast-feed.

Fluid intake

Approximately ninety per cent of breast milk is water. It is therefore essential that you drink enough fluid. It must be pointed out, however, that if you drink too much, this will not cause a further increase in the amount of milk you produce. The excess water will simply be passed out as urine. While you ensure that you drink enough, you must remember that you gain nothing by drinking too much fluid. It is sufficient to drink so that you are never thirsty; this usually means about two or three pints (1-1½ litres) per day.

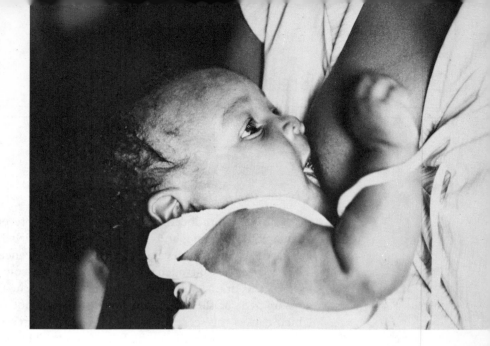

Fig 3.1
Suckling causes the breast to produce more milk.

Breast-feeding

The actual process of the baby suckling from the breasts makes them produce more milk. Our ancestors were aware of this fact and tried to use it when rearing motherless babies. These babies were suckled on their grandmothers' breasts. Unfortunately, milk produced by these elderly women was not sufficient for the babies' needs! Emptying the breasts completely during feeding also makes them produce more milk. Failure to empty the breasts may cause a reduction in the amount of milk they produce. If this persists, the breasts may stop producing milk altogether.

State of mind

We often forget that our state of mind has a profound influence on the activities of our brain. Some brain activities are more influenced than others. The secretion of breast milk is one of the brain activities which is affected by our state of mind. If you are anxious, afraid or unhappy, you may eventually produce little or no milk. For example, mothers in war-affected areas are sometimes unable to produce enough milk for their babies.

Severe illness

Occasionally, severe illness in a nursing mother causes the supply of breast milk to fail or to be drastically reduced. In most cases, this does not matter very much because breast-feeding is not usually advisable if the nursing mother is seriously ill.

If your baby is too ill to suck from the breast, your breasts will tend to dry up unless you take the precaution of squeezing and emptying them as soon as they fill up.

The composition of breast milk

Milk is the only complete food in nature. This is not surprising since young mammals depend entirely on their mothers' milk for nourishment. Like all balanced diets, breast milk contains carbohydrates such as lactose, protein, fat, vitamins and minerals. It also contains plenty of water. The concentration and quality of the main food constituents are shown in Fig 3.2.

	Percentage concentration	Quality
Carbohydrate	7.0%	Easily digested
Fat	3.5%	Fine particles High quality Easily digested
Protein	1.5%	High quality Easily digested

Fig 3.2   The main food constituents of breast milk.

The protein in breast milk includes **antibodies**. These are extremely important in the battle against disease and protect young infants against many types of infection. This is one of the reasons why breast-feeding is so important for newborn babies.

The fat in breast milk is easily digested and absorbed by young babies.

Some vitamins, especially vitamins B and C, are not stored in the human body. For this reason, the quantity of vitamins present in your breast milk depends on the quantity in your diet while you are breast-feeding. You should therefore make sure that you eat enough meat, fish, fruit and vegetables.

Colostrum

The milk which you produce in the first week following your confinement is known as **colostrum**. It is especially rich, particularly in protein. It should therefore be fed to the baby rather than squeezed out and thrown away. It is sometimes yellowish in colour and may leave a yellowish stain on your underclothes. Your baby may have frequent bowel motions while feeding on colostrum but he will continue to gain weight. *You should not regard these frequent bowel motions as diarrhoea.*

Drugs affecting breast milk

Certain drugs which you may take can pass into your breast milk after entering into your bloodstream. Some of these drugs are:
a) antibiotics such as penicillin, tetracycline and chloramphenicol;
b) pain-killing drugs such as aspirin and paracetamol (or Panadol);
c) sleeping tablets such as barbiturates and bromides;
d) strong laxatives, the majority of which can pass into breast milk;
e) alcohol and
f) nicotine in cigarette smoke.

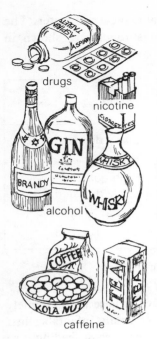

drugs

nicotine

alcohol

caffeine

Some drugs may be harmful to your baby especially if large quantities are present in your breast milk. For example, *tetracycline* (also known as Terramycin) can hamper the growth of your baby's teeth and bones. *Aspirin* can cause **jaundice** in newborn babies.

Alcohol enters into breast milk very easily. If present in large amounts, it can affect your baby's brain and cause convulsions. You must not drink many alcoholic drinks during the period when you are breast-feeding.

Nicotine is another drug which enters into breast milk easily. It is the main drug in cigarette smoke and can damage your baby's brain. You should not smoke more than two or three cigarettes a day while you are breast-feeding. Since it is usually easier to give up smoking than to cut it down, it is probably better for you to stop smoking altogether until you have stopped breast-feeding.

Tea, coffee and kola nuts contain *caffeine* which is a brain stimulant. This is why people chew kola nuts or drink strong coffee when they wish to stay awake at night. Fortunately, caffeine does not pass into breast milk easily. However, you should avoid drinking large amounts of tea or coffee or chewing kola nuts in the late afternoon and evening. This is because your breast milk may then contain enough caffeine to keep your baby awake all night.

Preparing for breast-feeding

If you look closely at your baby while breast-feeding, you will notice that the whole length of your nipple is inside your baby's mouth while his lips are grasping the dark portion of your breast just beyond the nipple. This dark area is known as the **areola**. Obviously, if your breast is dirty or infected, it is very easy for the dirt or infection to enter your baby's mouth and digestive tract. It is therefore important that your breasts are clean and free from rashes or other infections *at all times*. For this reason you should always wash your breast with a little soap and water before you breast-feed.

Fig 3.3
Position of the baby's lips during breast-feeding.

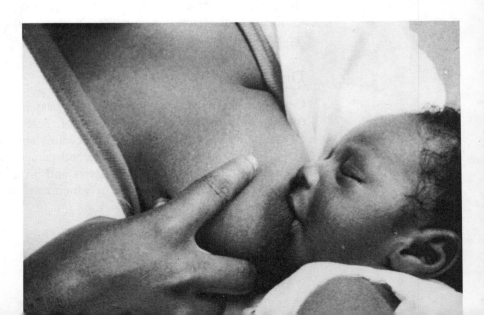

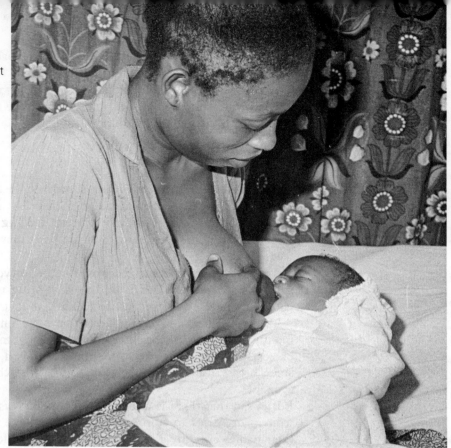

Fig 3.4
The mother should adopt
a comfortable position
for breast-feeding.

When you are ready to start breast-feeding, you should adopt a position which you find comfortable. Your baby's head should be cradled in the crook of your arm while you support his body in a reclining position. It is not, however, advisable for your baby to lie completely flat during breast-feeding as regurgitation can occur more easily in this position.

Methods

There are two methods of breast-feeding. These are feeding on schedule and feeding on demand.

Feeding on schedule

This is the method which is often adopted in developed countries. The baby is fed every four hours, starting at 6.00 a.m. and ending at 10.00 p.m. Babies under three months of age may require an additional night feed at 2.00 a.m.

When feeding on schedule, the nursing mother should possess a clock in her home by which she can tell the time.

Feeding on demand

This method is more popular in developing countries. The baby is fed whenever he cries for food. Since many African mothers still carry their babies on their backs, their breast milk is constantly available and their

25

babies' cries can be readily answered. Most babies establish their own schedule which is often not very different from the four-hourly schedule.

The disadvantage of feeding on demand is that a lazy or sickly baby may not feed often enough. Also, it may not be easy to tell whether a baby is crying from hunger or for some other reason.

Duration

Most of the milk in your breast is emptied in the first five minutes of suckling. However, ten minutes on each breast is usually recommended which brings the total duration of breast-feeding to twenty minutes. It is important to note that a slow or sickly baby may take longer than this to feed.

After your baby has suckled from one breast you may hold him up and rub his back gently. This is said to help bring up any wind which your baby may have swallowed while suckling, but it is not essential.

Ideally, you should breast-feed your baby until he is at least twelve months old. In developing countries, many mothers breast-feed their babies for more than twelve months. This is a good practice especially since breast milk is such a good source of rich protein and is readily available.

It is sad that there is a tendency for an increasing number of educated women in Africa to stop breast-feeding for one reason or another when their babies are only a few months old. They then feed their babies with artificial milk instead. As we shall see in the next chapter, feeding babies with artificial milk can have its own problems.

Advantages and disadvantages

Breast milk has several advantages.
1. It is rich and easily digested.
2. It does not have to be purchased.
3. It is available at all times.
4. It does not need to be specially prepared.
5. It is produced at the right temperature.
6. It does not contain harmful germs.
7. It contains antibodies which protect the baby against many infections.

Breast-feeding also has the advantage that it promotes a close bond between mother and baby and is emotionally satisfying for both mother and baby.

The only disadvantage of breast-feeding is that it puts a strain on the mother. If she is eating well she need not worry about this strain but breast-feeding is not advisable if the mother is seriously ill. Should a mother who is breast-feeding become pregnant again, she should stop breast-feeding as she could not then afford the double strain of pregnancy and breast-feeding.

Complications

There are only a few complications which may arise from breast-feeding. Of these, cracked nipples, breast engorgement, breast abscesses and debility are the only notable ones.

Cracked nipples

Occasionally, the skin around the nipple cracks and becomes painful. The pain increases when the baby is actually feeding and so the nursing mother becomes reluctant to feed her baby with the affected breast. The breast subsequently becomes engorged causing extra pain. Resting the breast for a day and painting the nipple with gentian violet is usually sufficient treatment to heal the nipple. The breast should be gently squeezed to prevent engorgement. Always ensure that your nipple is placed well inside your baby's mouth to avoid injury from your baby's teeth.

Breast engorgement

This is caused by the breast becoming too full of milk. It is a painful condition which occurs most often as a complication of cracked nipples. It can be treated by gently squeezing the breast although this may be painful and difficult. If it is not relieved in time, engorgement may be followed by the suppression of milk production which is clearly not desirable in normal circumstances.

Breast abscesses

The neglect of a cracked nipple may lead to infection and hence to the formation of an abscess within the breast. This is a serious complication which requires prompt treatment with antibiotics. If an abscess forms, it should also be drained promptly.

Debility

A nursing mother who does not eat enough may become debilitated from breast-feeding. If she was already undernourished before she started breast-feeding her baby, she may become dangerously debilitated.

If the mother is nursing twins (or on rare occasions triplets) she must take extra care to eat enough nourishing food (also see page 33). In the past, as result of poverty and ignorance about balanced diets, mothers of twins often died from anaemia and malnutrition.

Unsuccessful breast-feeding

Breast-feeding may be unsuccessful for various reasons including:
a) the inadequate production of breast milk;
b) flat or retracted nipples which prevent the baby from suckling and
c) a severe illness or deformity in the baby which makes it difficult or impossible for the baby to feed from the breast.

In (b) and (c) the continued production of milk soon causes the breast to become engorged and painful. This can be prevented by giving the mother a short course of treatment with an appropriate drug to suppress further milk production.

4 | Bottle-feeding

Artificial milk

All milk other than breast milk is known as artificial milk and can be the milk from cows, goats, buffaloes or camels. Milk from all these animals has been used in feeding babies at some time in different parts of the world. Feeding babies with artificial milk is known as artificial feeding. Cows' milk is by far the most commonly used. The composition and quality of the main constituents of cows' milk are shown in Fig 4.1.

	Percentage concentration	Quality
Carbohydrate	4.5%	Same as in breast milk
Protein	3.5%	Poor quality Difficult to digest
Fat	3.5%	Coarse particles Difficult to digest

Fig 4.1   The main food constituents of cows' milk.

Cows' milk contains less carbohydrate than breast milk. It contains more protein but of a lower quality which is difficult for human babies to digest. The stringy material which is frequently found in the faeces of babies fed on cows' milk is caused by undigested cows' milk protein.

Cows' milk contains the same amount of fat as breast milk but this fat is in form of coarse particles which are tough and difficult to digest.

Cows' milk contains fewer vitamins and more minerals than breast milk. The kidneys of human babies find it difficult to deal with the relatively large amounts of minerals in cows' milk. These minerals cause calcium to collect in the infant's intestines and so reduce the amount of calcium absorbed into the body, in which case the baby may become short of calcium. If persistent this shortage of calcium can hamper the proper development of the bones. In addition, the baby may become jittery and may develop convulsions.

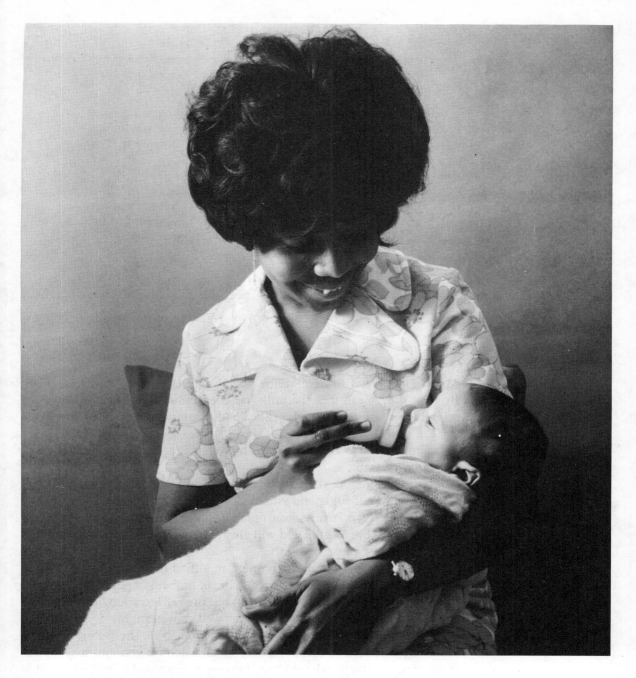

Fig 4.2   Bottle-feeding.

Lastly, cows' milk does not contain antibodies which, as we have seen, are important for protecting babies against infection. Infants fed only on cows' milk are very liable to suffer from all sorts of infection. The differences between cows' milk and breast milk are summarised in Fig 4.3.

	Breast milk		Cows' milk	
Carbohydrate	7.0%	Good quality	4.5%	Good quality
Fat	3.5%	Fine particles Easily digested	3.5%	Coarse particles Congeals easily Difficult to digest
Protein	1.5%	High quality Easily digested	3.5%	Poor quality Difficult to digest
Vitamins		Present in appreciable quantities		Not present in sufficient quantities
Minerals		Not too many		Too many
Antibodies		Present		Absent

Fig 4.3   Differences between cows' milk and breast milk.

Modified cows' milk

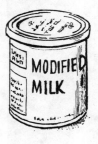

Many commercial firms describe their brand of cows' milk as modified. By this, they mean that the milk has been modified in such a way as to resemble breast milk closely. The modification process has three basic stages:

a) boiling—to break up and soften the tough protein and coarse fat particles in cows' milk;

b) dilution—to reduce the concentration of protein and minerals and

c) the addition of sugar and vitamins.

Unfortunately, no matter how much it is modified, cows' milk cannot be converted into breast milk and will always be different from breast milk as far as babies are concerned.

Powdered milk is the most common modified milk preparation used in infant-feeding in African countries. This is probably because the powder keeps well in hot weather and does not require refrigeration. The tins have closely fitting lids which are airtight as well as watertight.

Dried or powdered milk is milk from which all the water has been removed. It is sold in tins of various sizes. Each tin contains a scoop for measuring out the powder. Instructions for preparing the feeds are written on the tin and must be followed carefully as different brands have different instructions. When reconstituted according to the instructions, this milk contains the same number of calories per ounce as breast milk.

Several brands of modified powdered milk are available in the markets. They are all described as 'modified' on the tin and there is little difference between the individual brands. Some brands have the words 'full-cream' or 'half-cream' written on the tin. Full-cream means that the powder contains the full complement of fat whereas half-cream means that the powder contains only half the amount of fat present in the same quantity of full-cream milk. Half-cream is used mainly in feeding newborn babies who are unable to tolerate the quantity of fat in normal or full-cream milk. Half-cream powdered milk is not imported into many African countries.

Unmodified cows' milk

Dried milk

Several types of unmodified cows' milk are available, the most common being dried, evaporated, condensed, skimmed and boiled fresh milk. However, only some of these are suitable for infant-feeding.

Modified dried milk has already been mentioned but *ordinary dried milk for kitchen use must not be confused with the modified variety*. The dried milk will not be modified unless it is stated on the tin and unmodified dried milk is not suitable for bottle-feeding young infants although it may be used to make up weaning foods for older infants.

Evaporated milk

Evaporated milk contains half the quantity of water present in fresh milk. It is therefore twice as concentrated as fresh milk and has to be diluted with an equal amount of water to reconstitute it.

Evaporated milk is usually sold in small tins under various brand names and is used mainly for preparing beverages. Some mothers also use it for preparing pap and other similar foods for weaning their infants but *it is not suitable for bottle-feeding babies of less than six months*.

The disadvantage of evaporated milk is that once the tin has been opened the milk does not keep for more than a few days, even when the tin is kept in a refrigerator.

Condensed milk

Condensed milk is ten times more concentrated than fresh milk. It is sold in tins and keeps longer than evaporated milk but not as well as powdered milk. It must be used up as quickly as possible once the tin has been opened. It is not popular in African countries and is not easily available.

A considerable amount of sugar is sometimes added during the preparation of condensed milk and if so the product is then known as *sweetened* condensed milk. *It is not suitable for infant-feeding*.

Skimmed milk

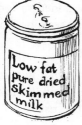

Skimmed milk is fat-free powdered milk. It is usually available in bags. Large quantities have, in the past, been imported into Africa but, as some people discovered, it can cause diarrhoea in both children and adults.

Skimmed milk is used mainly for feeding whole communities which are deficient in protein but *it is not at all suitable for infant-feeding* except in very rare cases where the infant cannot tolerate milk fat. In such a case, the infant's fat requirements would be provided in the form of cod-liver oil.

Boiled fresh milk

In Africa, fresh cows' milk is not readily available in many regions. Because of this, boiled milk is sometimes imported in large bottles and sold in the big departmental stores.

Unboiled cows' milk should not be used to feed babies. Firstly, it is often contaminated by germs, the most dangerous of which are tuberculosis germs. Secondly, as was previously mentioned, babies cannot easily digest

Fig 4.4
Preparing fresh cows'
milk for bottle-feeding.

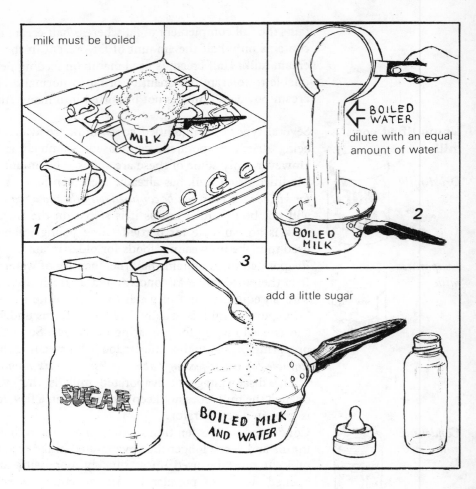

the protein and fat in unboiled cows' milk. To make it safe and more digestible, *cows' milk must be boiled before use*. It is also advisable to dilute it with an equal amount of water in order to reduce the concentration of protein and minerals. A little sugar should then be added to increase the sugar content which otherwise would be too low. One teaspoonful of sugar per feed will be sufficient for this (see Fig 4.4).

All the milk preparations described above, except fresh cows' milk, have been subjected to heat and are free of germs. Contamination, therefore, can only occur as a result of careless handling by the user.

Choosing the brand of milk

Powdered, modified milk is suitable for use in the tropics. It is the preparation preferred by African mothers. There is very little difference between the different brands of powdered milk. The cheaper brands are just as good as the expensive ones. It is sensible to try to keep to a brand which suits your baby but, if that brand is not available for some reason, it will do no harm to try another brand.

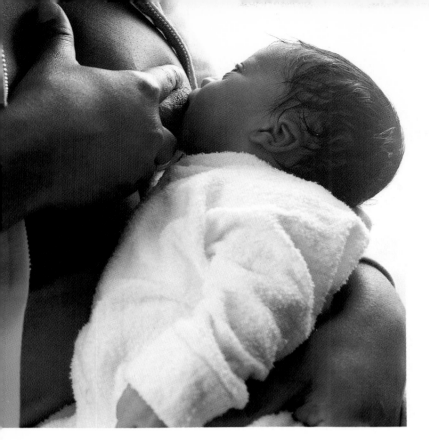

Breast-feeding

Breast-feeding is the best way to make your baby healthy and strong. The nipples should be washed, rinsed and dried before each feed. Always wash your hands before putting your baby to the breast (see Chapter 3).

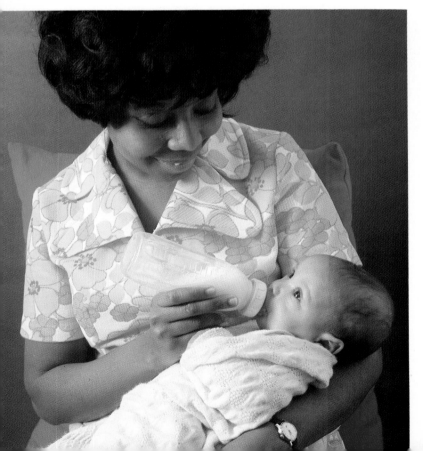

Bottle-feeding

If you are bottle-feeding your baby, either to supplement breast-feeding or because you have been advised to do so, you must *always* use correctly prepared artificial milk which has been modified for this purpose (see Chapter 4).

Colour plate 1

Bathing

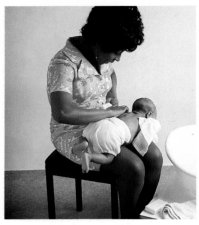

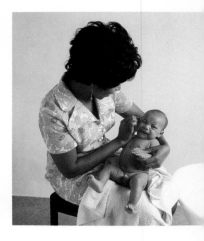

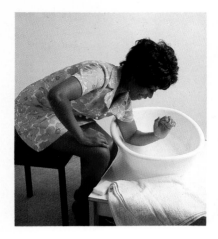

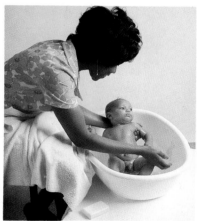

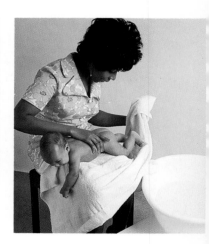

The baby should be bathed every day in clean, warm water. Pour warm water into a tub or basin and test the temperature with your elbow.

Undress the baby on your lap, holding him firmly.

Clean his face gently with a dampened face towel or cotton wool. Carefully wipe his eyes, nose and ears.

Soap the hair gently with your hand, then rinse carefully and pat dry with a towel.

Carefully soap his body, avoiding his face. Then lower him gently into the water, holding his head up, and always holding his body firmly. Let him splash to wash off the soap.

Now place him on a towel on your lap and wrap him in the towel to dry him gently. Make sure to dry in the creases — under the arms, between the legs and around the neck.

Colour plate 2

terilising the bottle by boiling

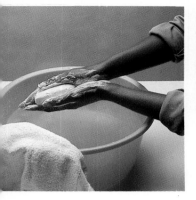

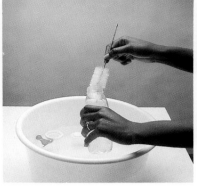

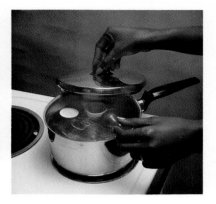

'ash your hands.

Rinse the bottle, caps and teats in clean, cold water. Then wash with detergent using a bottle-brush. Then rinse again in clean water.

Place the bottle and caps in a pan, cover with clean water and boil for ten minutes. Add the teats and boil for another three minutes. Leave in the sterilised water with a lid on the pan until you prepare the next feed (see also Chapter 4 for the method using sterilising solution).

eeping your baby clean

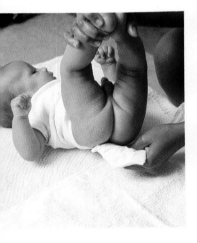

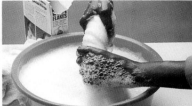

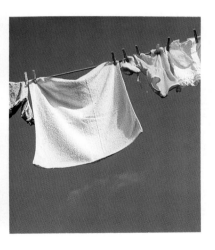

lean your baby with something oft whenever he is wet or dirty nd change his nappy if he is earing one.
ake sure that he is dry and omfortable before you feed him lie him down to sleep.

Soiled nappies must be rinsed off and soaked immediately. They should then be washed, rinsed and hung out to dry (see Chapter 6).

Clothing should be washed frequently and dried in the sun.

Clothing for hot weather

Babies need very little clothing in hot weather. Their clothing should be light and loose fitting (see Chapter 6).

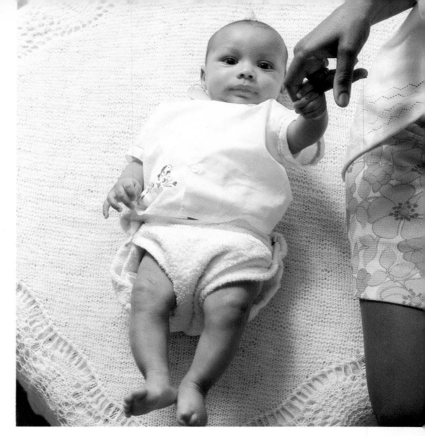

Clothing for cool weather

Babies become cold very easily and so need extra clothing at night and on cool days (see Chapter 6). You could also wrap your baby in a blanket and keep him close to you.

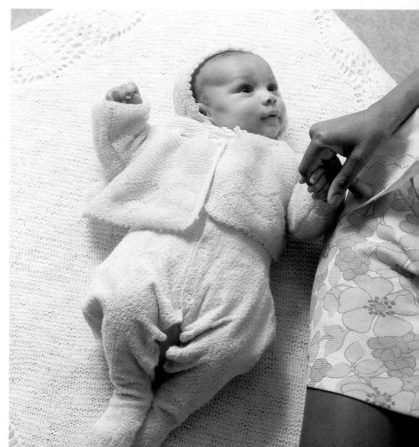

Colour plate 4

Common reasons for bottle-feeding

There are many reasons for bottle-feeding; these are some of the most common ones.

1. *Inadequacy or failure of breast-feeding*
   The reasons for this have been discussed in Chapter 3.
2. *Employment of the mother outside the home*
   Many working mothers cannot take their infants with them when they go to work. This means that the infants have to be bottle-fed by the baby's nurse while the mother is away, although the mother could still breast-feed when she is at home.
3. *Multiple births such as twins or triplets*
   In such cases, where the mother's breast milk may be inadequate for the babies' growth, bottle-feeding is usually recommended in addition to breast-feeding.
4. *Pregnancy*
   As was mentioned in Chapter 3, a nursing mother who becomes pregnant should stop breast-feeding if she feels that the combined strain of

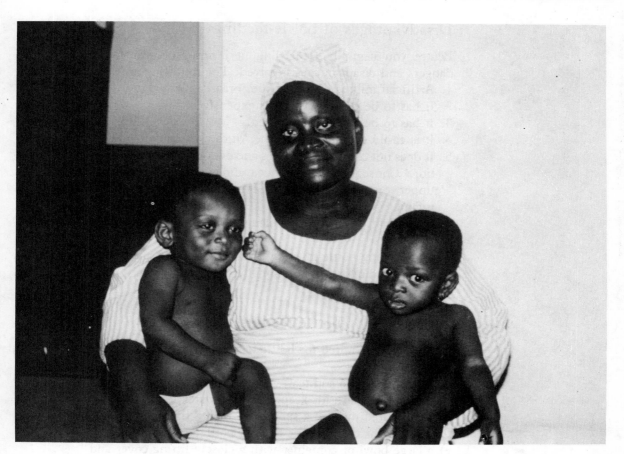

Fig 4.5   In the case of twins, the mother's milk may not be adequate.

breast-feeding and pregnancy is becoming too much for her. She should try to increase her intake of food to overcome this.

5. *Refusal of the breast*

Occasionally an infant will, of his own accord, refuse to feed from the breast. This happens most often when the infant has been fed with a brand of powdered milk which contains more sugar than breast milk. The infant then prefers the sweeter artificial milk to breast milk. Sometimes, however, there are other reasons for the refusal of the breast, such as an inverted nipple.

6. *Aversion to breast-feeding*

Some mothers, consciously or unconsciously, dislike breast-feeding. This aversion may be openly expressed in more developed countries but it is usually hidden behind more acceptable reasons in developing countries. It is interesting to note that most mothers bottle-feed their infants from choice and not because of any of the reasons listed above. They start bottle-feeding needlessly because they have been persuaded by advertising that artificial feeding is particularly good for their infants.

Disadvantages of bottle-feeding

Before you begin bottle-feeding, it is important for you to know the dangers and disadvantages involved. The following are some of them.
1. Artificial milk is different from breast milk.
2. It has to be purchased and is expensive.
3. It has to be carefully prepared.
4. It is easily contaminated either during storage or preparation.
5. It does not contain antibodies and does not protect infants against infection. Consequently, diarrhoea and vomiting, urinary infections and upper respiratory tract infections are more common in bottle-fed infants.
6. It can cause digestive problems in infants who cannot tolerate cows' milk.
7. The feeding bottle must be carefully sterilised and kept free of germs.
8. Bottle-feeding is less emotionally satisfying for both mother and baby.

Preparing for bottle-feeding

The utensils required for bottle-feeding, which are illustrated in Fig 4.6, are:
a) a feeding bottle and teat;
b) a Thermos flask for keeping boiled water;
c) a calibrated jug and a spoon for mixing the milk;
d) a brush for cleaning the feeding bottle;
e) a large bowl or container with a closely fitting cover and
f) sterilising solution, if the bottle and teat cannot be sterilised by boiling.

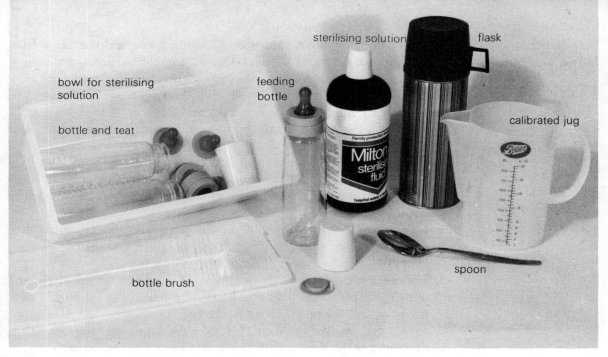

Fig 4.6 Utensils for bottle-feeding and sterilising equipment.

Feeding bottles

Feeding bottles are available in various sizes. At one time they were all made of glass but plastic ones are now available and easy to acquire. Glass bottles are easier to keep clean and can be sterilised easily by boiling but they are breakable. Plastic ones do not break but generally cannot withstand boiling and are therefore more difficult to sterilise. There are good quality plastic bottles now available which can be boiled but only if this is clearly stated.

You can begin by buying only one feeding bottle and then you can always buy more if necessary. Some feeding bottles have lids which cover and protect the teat. These are very useful for travelling.

Teats are now made from synthetic rubber. They resemble and function like the mother's nipple. However, unlike the mother's nipple which has several holes, teats have only one hole out of which the milk flows.

Teats can have holes of various sizes. You must be careful to choose one with a suitable hole. If the hole is too small, the infant has to suck very hard and may become tired before he has got enough milk. He may also swallow a lot of air in the process. If the hole is too big, the milk will come out too quickly and may choke the infant. The best way to tell whether or not the hole is adequate, is to test how quickly the milk comes out of the bottle. It should come out in rapid drops and not in a continuous stream.

As a rule, teats tend to have holes that are too small. You can enlarge the hole using the blunt end of a large needle. This can be done by sticking the sharp end of the needle into a cork, then heating the blunt end until it is red hot, and pushing it quickly but gently into the hole in the teat.

35

Sterilising the bottle and teat

It is very important that your baby's feeding bottle and teat are sterile, meaning free of germs, at all times. One method for sterilising and boiling is illustrated on colour plate 3, but since many feeding bottles are now made of plastic, they cannot be sterilised by boiling. However, they can be kept sterile by using the following measures.

1. After each feed, wash out the bottle with a brush, soap and water. Use the brush to clean away all the milk particles.
2. Rinse thoroughly to remove all traces of soap.
3. Sprinkle ordinary table salt on the teat and clean it by rubbing it between your fingers. Then rinse it with water which has been boiled to ensure that it is really clean.
4. Prepare some sterilising solution (Milton) using boiled water in a large bowl or container as directed on the bottle. Change the solution daily.
5. Fill the feeding bottle with the prepared sterilising solution, put the teat on the bottle and immerse bottle and teat in the solution. Cover the bowl with its lid and keep it covered.
6. When you prepare the next feed, take the bottle and teat out of the bowl, pour out the sterilising solution and rinse in clean water.

Clean water

Clean water comes mainly in the form of pipe-borne water. Unfortunately, some homes do not have access to pipe-borne water and instead water from streams, wells, rivers or ponds is used. The water you use for preparing your baby's feed, and for preparing the sterilising solution, must be boiled for at least *ten minutes* to ensure that it is really clean. If there is any sediment it usually settles at the bottom as the water is allowed to cool. The clear water above the sediment should be poured directly into the flask or sterilising bowl. It should not be transferred with a cup or bowl as contamination may take place in the process. It may be safer to avoid bottle-feeding altogether when clean pipe-borne water is not available.

Preparing the feed

The instructions for preparing the feeds are always written clearly on the tin. *You must follow these instructions very carefully*. Fig 4.7 is taken from a tin of one of the popular brands of powdered modified milk.

As you can see from Fig 4.7, the amount of feed required by your baby increases as your baby grows older. If you do not understand the instructions on the tin, you must ask someone who can to help you.

Your baby may require slightly more or slightly less than the amount recommended by the manufacturers. This is sometimes stated on the tin. If your baby finishes his feed at each meal, you may have to offer him a little more than is recommended.

You must wash your hands thoroughly before preparing the feed and also make sure that your fingers do not touch the milk powder or the water used for mixing the milk.

Average Age	Average weight (kg)	No. of feeds per day	Level scoops of powder	Made up with boiled water (ml)
Newborn	2.5 (5½ lb)	6	2 to 3	85 (3 fl.oz.)
2 weeks	3.4 (7½ lb)	6	2 to 3	85 (3 fl.oz.)
1 month	3.9 (8½ lb)	6	3 to 4	85 to 110 (3 to 4 fl.oz.)
2 months	4.8 (10½ lb)	6	4	115 (4 fl.oz.)
3 months	5.7 (12½ lb)	5	6	170 (6 fl.oz.)
4 months	6.3 (14lb)	5	6 to 7	170 to 200 (6 to 7 fl.oz.)
5 months	7.0 (15½ lb)	5	7 to 8	200 to 230 (7 to 8 fl.oz.)
6 months and over	7.7 (17lb)	5	8	230 (8 fl.oz.)

Fig 4.7   A typical feeding table for powdered milk feeds.

When preparing the feed, place the number of scoops of milk recommended in the calibrated jug. Then add the appropriate amount of boiled water and mix thoroughly with a spoon until there are *no* lumps in the feed. After mixing, pour the mixed milk *carefully* into the feeding bottle, being careful to leave out any milk sediment (see Fig 4.8).

Fig 4.8
Preparing a powdered milk feed.

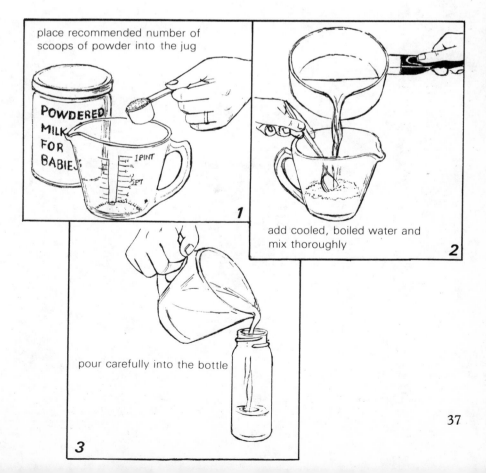

place recommended number of scoops of powder into the jug

POWDERED MILK FOR BABIES

1

add cooled, boiled water and mix thoroughly

2

pour carefully into the bottle

3

Feeding with a cup and spoon

Because some mothers find it difficult to keep the feeding bottle and teat sterile, some doctors are of the opinion that a cup and spoon are safer, as these are much easier to keep clean. However, feeding a small infant using a cup and spoon is a slow and tedious process. The decision to recommend a cup and spoon instead of a feeding bottle will depend on the circumstances in individual cases.

Hygiene in the home

The importance of hygiene

There are many causes of illness which can affect human beings. These can be divided into five main groups:

a) infections, causing such things as boils, pneumonia and dysentery;
b) lack of substances vital for life, such as food or air;
c) degeneration or ageing of the body organs;
d) injury or poisoning, and
e) tumours such as those causing cancer.

Infections are by far the most common causes of illness. They cause more illness than all the other four groups together. They are spread by harmful organisms.

The main reason for observing hygiene in the home is to prevent infection by reducing the number of harmful organisms in the home.

Harmful organisms

All living creatures are organisms which share many of the same basic characteristics such as growth, reproduction and feeding. Harmful organisms include pests and parasites, such as worms, which can be seen with the naked eye. However the most harmful organisms are so tiny that they can only be seen with the help of a microscope. These are known as **micro-organisms** or microbes. The four main types of harmful micro-organisms are bacteria, viruses, protozoa and fungi. Infections caused by bacteria and viruses are more common than those caused by protozoa and fungi. Harmful micro-organisms are often known as germs. Some viruses are so tiny that they cannot be seen with an ordinary microscope and can only be viewed with the help of a special high-powered electron microscope.

Micro-organisms are present all around us, in the air we breathe, on the clothes we wear, and on the walls and furniture in our homes.

If food is left exposed for some days, it soon becomes covered with mould. This mould is caused by the micro-organisms which are present in the air.

Micro-organisms are also present in the human body particularly on the skin, especially around the groin and the anus, in the upper air passages, especially the nostrils, in the mouth and throat, and in the lower parts of the digestive tract, including the large bowel and anus.

| **Favourable conditions for growth** | Like all living creatures, micro-organisms thrive under certain conditions. Some of the more important of these are discussed here. |

Warmth

A warm climate favours the growth of micro-organisms, so people in the tropics have to be especially careful to control the number of micro-organisms in the environment.

Micro-organisms do not grow at all in a very cold environment. This is why food does not decay rapidly when it is kept in a good refrigerator.

Moisture

All living creatures require water, or at least moisture, to stay alive. Micro-organisms do not thrive in a dry environment.

Darkness

Dark places are also likely to be moist and dirty and so might harbour micro-organisms. Some micro-organisms cannot live at all in the presence of air and light and so are more likely to be found in dark places. Dark corners inside the house should be swept regularly as insects also tend to collect there.

Dirt and decay

Many organisms, particularly micro-organisms, live by breaking down rotting waste organic matter. Dirt containing organic matter such as waste food or other kitchen refuse, faeces and urine harbour micro-organisms as well as larger pests such as flies and rats.

Overcrowding

Homes which are overcrowded with people or their belongings are extremely difficult to keep clean. Such homes contain many dark corners which provide good hiding places for pests and organisms.

Bad personal habits

If we cough or sneeze without covering our mouths and nostrils we expel many micro-organisms from our air passages into the surrounding atmosphere. The same thing happens if we spit on the ground. The result is that the air around us becomes polluted with these micro-organisms.

Whenever we go to the toilet our fingers pick up more micro-organisms. Therefore, unless we wash our hands immediately after going to the toilet, we invariably spread the micro-organisms to whatever we then touch with our fingers.

Pests

The household pests which are commonly found in homes in the tropics are flies, mosquitoes, cockroaches, and rats. These pests play a very important part in spreading infections. This fact is often forgotten or ignored by many of us.

Pests spread infections in many ways. They carry dangerous micro-organisms on their hairy legs and spread these micro-organisms from place to place. They are frequently deposited on food. Flies are the most notorious pests in this respect. Many pests, such as rats and cockroaches, deposit their excreta on the floor and on food, making it unsafe to eat. Gari is often contaminated in this way. Excreta also acts as food for flies and micro-organisms, so allowing them to thrive. Food poisoning (**salmonella**) and lung infection (**leptospirosis**) are examples of diseases spread by

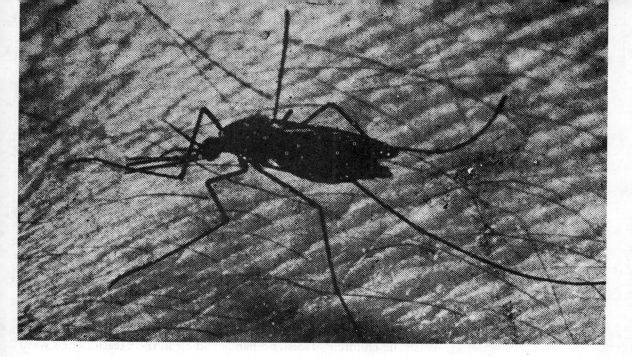

Fig 5.1   A mosquito is a common household pest in the tropics.

vermin excreta. An insect may suck fluid from an infected person and then inject this infection into the next healthy person it feeds on. Mosquitoes spread malaria infection in this way.

Domestic animals

The domestic animals most commonly found in tropical areas are chickens, goats, sheep and cows. There are also pets, mainly cats and dogs.

Although cats and dogs are usually clean in their habits, this cannot be said to be true for the other animals. Some people allow chickens and goats to enter the house and, as a result, animal excreta litters the floor and makes the home very unhealthy. **Toxocara canis**, tetanus, **brucellosis** and tapeworm are some of the diseases spread by domestic animals.

The compound, as well as the floors inside the house, should be swept daily and all animal excreta buried. This is because children play in the compound and may catch diseases if the compound is not kept clean.

Harmful micro-organisms

Harmful micro-organisms can enter the body through the air we breathe, in our food or drink and through our skin.

Some of the common infections which are spread by breathing contaminated air include the common cold, bronchitis, pneumonia, measles, whooping cough and tuberculosis.

Infections which are spread through contaminated food or drink include all the diarrhoeal diseases, worms, infective hepatitis, typhoid fever and dysentery.

Skin infections (such as scabies (craw-craw), boils and ringworm), tetanus and hookworm anaemia are examples of infections spread through the skin.

Cleanliness and daily routine

We now know the conditions which favour the growth and spread of harmful micro-organisms, as well as how harmful organisms enter the human body. If we wish to avoid infections we must observe strict cleanliness in our daily routine. The following daily routine is meant only as a guide.

1. Every morning on waking up, open all windows to let in fresh air and sunlight.
2. Sweep all the rooms and the compound and bury all refuse.
3. Dust all the furniture.
4. Wash the children's faces and hands and clean their teeth. Then wash your own face and hands and clean your own teeth.
5. Prepare the breakfast, remembering that all food left over from the previous evening should be boiled before eating.
6. Serve the food immediately after it has been cooked. Never leave food exposed to dust and flies.
7. Prepare and serve afternoon and evening meals in the same manner.
8. After preparing the evening meal, give the children a bath, clean their teeth, and then have a bath yourself before you have your meal.

Kitchen hygiene

Apart from malaria, diarrhoea is the most common cause of illness in children. Many of these cases of diarrhoea occur because strict hygiene has not been observed in the kitchen.

The kitchen is the most important room in the house as far as hygiene is concerned. Unfortunately, conditions in many kitchens encourage the spread of micro-organisms. The kitchen is usually the smallest and most overcrowded room in the house. Sometimes it is no more than a shed. It is often infested with flies during the day and with cockroaches and rats at night. It often serves as the sleeping quarters for domestic animals.

Cleanliness must be strictly observed in the kitchen. The following rules will help to reduce the spread of infection.

1. Wash your hands thoroughly before preparing a meal.
2. Wash up and tidy away after preparing each meal. Do not leave refuse and pieces of food lying about, particularly overnight. Always clean the work and food preparation surfaces, if necessary with disinfectant.
3. Never allow refuse to accumulate anywhere near your kitchen.

Hygiene in the compound

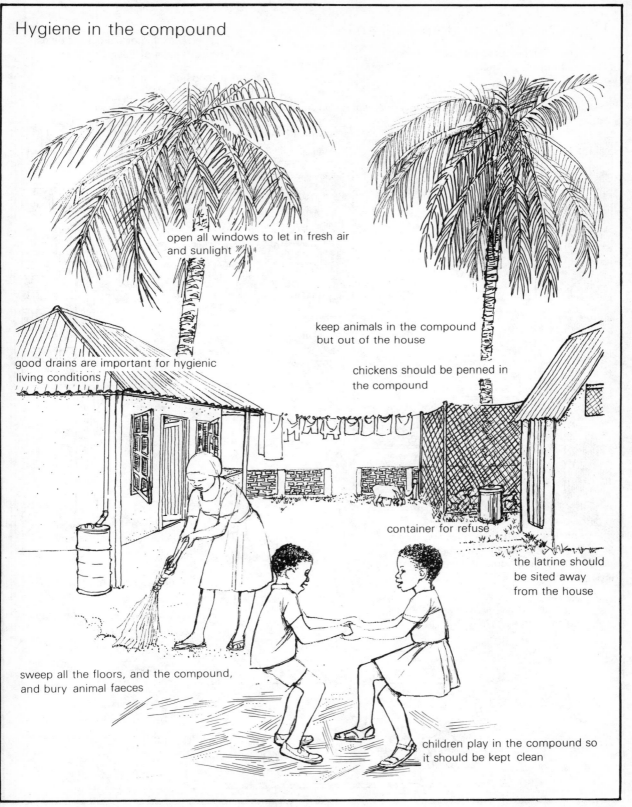

open all windows to let in fresh air and sunlight

keep animals in the compound but out of the house

chickens should be penned in the compound

good drains are important for hygienic living conditions

container for refuse

the latrine should be sited away from the house

sweep all the floors, and the compound, and bury animal faeces

children play in the compound so it should be kept clean

Hygiene in the modern kitchen

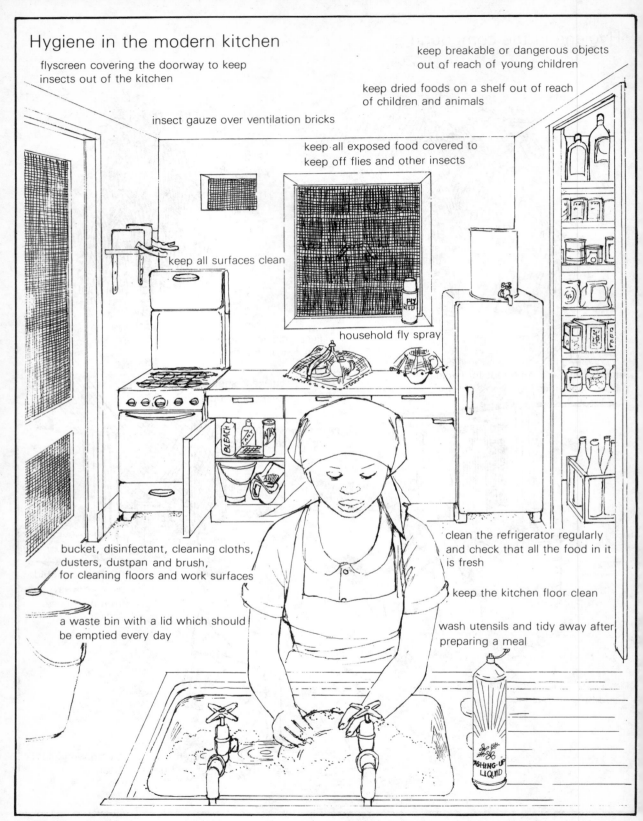

flyscreen covering the doorway to keep insects out of the kitchen

keep breakable or dangerous objects out of reach of young children

keep dried foods on a shelf out of reach of children and animals

insect gauze over ventilation bricks

keep all exposed food covered to keep off flies and other insects

keep all surfaces clean

household fly spray

bucket, disinfectant, cleaning cloths, dusters, dustpan and brush, for cleaning floors and work surfaces

clean the refrigerator regularly and check that all the food in it is fresh

keep the kitchen floor clean

a waste bin with a lid which should be emptied every day

wash utensils and tidy away after preparing a meal

Food item	In the pantry	In the refrigerator
Fresh meat and fish	1 day	2-3 days
Cooked food	Use immediately	1-2 days
		Boil thoroughly before eating
Tinned food (opened)	1 day	2-3 days
Frozen food (defrosted)	1 day	2-3 days
Vegetables and fruit	2-3 days, depending on ripeness	7-8 days, depending on ripeness

Fig 5.2　Times for which food items will stay fresh.

4. Always ensure that food is used before it goes bad. Fig 5.2 shows for approximately how long you can expect various foods to stay fresh. Food which has gone bad should be thrown away and must never be eaten.
5. Refrigerators should be cleaned out regularly with disinfectant and should be defrosted when necessary.
6. Do not let your baby soil your kitchen floor with urine or faeces as it is not at all easy to remove all traces of excreta from the floor.
7. Always wash your hands thoroughly after going to the toilet, and after changing your baby's nappy.

Bathing

In African countries, the weather is warm throughout the year except for short spells of cooler weather which occur during the harmattan and rainy seasons. As all mothers know, healthy children are very active and can play throughout the day. They usually play outside the house and so gather plenty of dirt in the process. Then, during the night, they perspire because of the warm weather. In view of this, children should be bathed at least once a day, usually before bedtime. The evening is a good time because bathing then washes away the dirt accumulated during the day and so does not allow it to cause infection.

Babies and small children should be bathed with mild toilet soap and a face towel. African soap is suitable but locally made bar soap is too strong and should not be used. African sponges should not be used because they are too rough and coarse for the delicate skin of small children (see also colour plate 2).

Failing to bath children adequately makes them more liable to develop skin infections. If your child is prone to skin infections (as some children

Hygiene in the modern bathroom

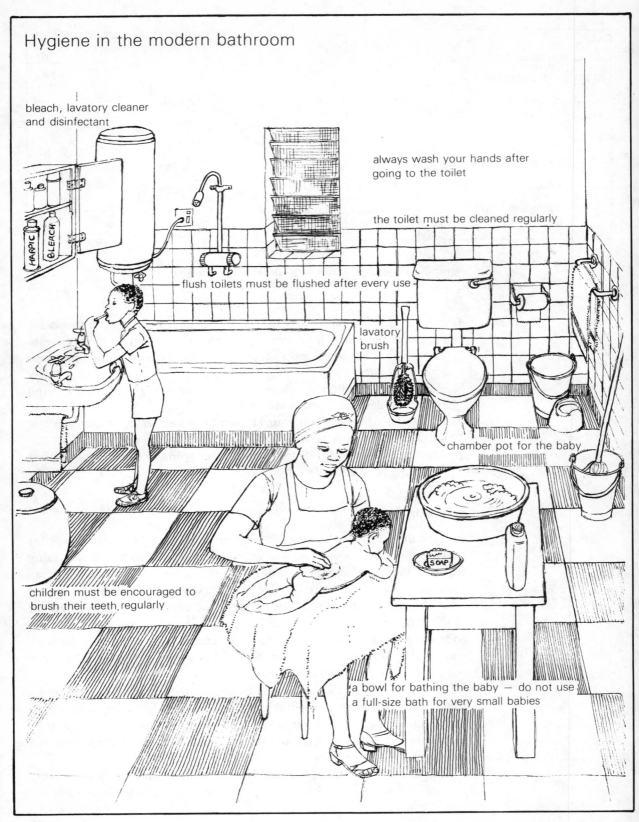

bleach, lavatory cleaner
and disinfectant

always wash your hands after
going to the toilet

the toilet must be cleaned regularly

flush toilets must be flushed after every use

lavatory
brush

chamber pot for the baby

children must be encouraged to
brush their teeth, regularly

a bowl for bathing the baby — do not use
a full-size bath for very small babies

are), ask a doctor to recommend a suitable antiseptic toilet soap which is available in your area.

Disposal of refuse

This is a very important factor to consider when trying to prevent the spread of disease. Refuse is disposed of in many ways, some of which are more hygienic than others. It should never be simply dumped at the back of the house, on street corners or thrown into nearby bushes, rivers or ponds. In some towns, refuse is collected from household dustbins by local council vans and then taken either to an incinerator or to a chosen piece of ground outside the town. In other towns, individual families are responsible for taking their own refuse to incinerators which are provided somewhere in the neighbourhood.

Refuse must always be buried or burned. It should never be left exposed for flies and other pests to thrive on. *If there is no refuse disposal service near your house, then you must dispose of your own refuse properly.*

Refuse dries quickly during the dry season and then can be easily disposed of by burning. During the rainy season, refuse is usually damp and will not then burn readily. Burying is therefore the easier method, particularly where there is enough ground in the compound. Buried refuse can then be used later as garden manure.

Disposal of faeces

Faeces can be disposed of in several ways, of which the following are the main ones.

Water-system, or flush, toilet

The most hygienic method of disposing of faeces *in areas where there is a dependable pipe-borne water supply* is by the water-system, or flush, method. However, this method is only hygienic if the toilet is flushed after every use and cleaned regularly with lavatory cleaner, or bleach, and a brush. If these precautions are not followed flush toilets can spread disease and are less hygienic than pit latrines. It is usually only homes which are in towns which possess water-system toilets because they have easier access to a dependable pipe-borne water supply.

Pit latrine

A deep pit latrine is the best means of faecal disposal if there is no dependable pipe-borne water supply. The pit should be at least six feet deep and three feet wide and should be sited as far away from the house as possible. Shallow pit latrines are as unhygienic as bucket latrines.

Pail or bucket

This is the most common method employed in many areas but unfortunately it is not at all a good method. The buckets are often not emptied regularly and are allowed to overflow. Flies and other pests have easy access to the faeces and carry micro-organisms from the buckets into homes.

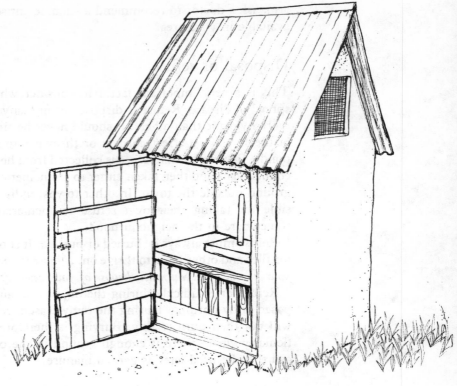

Fig 5.3
Latrine in the compound
away from the house.

Bushes, rivers or streams

Dumping faeces in bushes, rivers, streams or ponds is also unhygienic as it leaves the faeces exposed to the air and to flies. In addition, the water then becomes heavily contaminated and is therefore unsafe to use.

Drains

Many African homes lack good drains so that rain water, as well as dirty water from kitchens and bathrooms, is allowed to accumulate in the compound. The result is that flies, mosquitoes and other dangerous organisms are provided with a good breeding-ground. This is unhygienic for the people living in such homes and should be avoided at all costs. Every compound should be provided with good drains.

Summary

There are three main factors which promote good health and hygiene in the home. Firstly, the water which you use for cooking and drinking must be clean. If you are not sure that it is clean you should boil the water before you use it. Secondly, you must observe strict hygiene in the kitchen to ensure that you keep your food free from contamination. Thirdly, you must have proper latrine facilities and, whatever they may be, they should be cleaned regularly and dealt with in the appropriate manner.

48

6 Clothing for infants

It is quite common to see babies and young children wearing only a nappy or even without any clothes at all. Nudity in the very young is quite normal but at times it may be more sensible for young children to wear clothes.

The reasons for clothing infants are essentially the same as for clothing older children or adults. Clothes are worn not only for adornment but also to provide protection against unfavourable weather, insect bites and harmful organisms.

In African countries, the weather varies from season to season. You must ensure that, in the wet season, children have enough protection from the weather and an adequate supply of dry clothing. In the dry season, there may be some cool weather during which the children may need extra warmth, particularly at night. Before the rains, the weather may be very hot and humid and children should then have very light, cool clothing.

Types of clothing for infants

The following general guidelines may be useful when deciding on types of clothing for your infant. The clothing should be light, loose and easy to put on and take off. It should be easy to wash, be made of a material which does not irritate the skin but it must also be hard-wearing, otherwise the clothes will not last long in a tropical climate.

You may choose to make your infant's clothes yourself or to buy them from the market. In either case, it is useful to know something about the various types of clothing materials so that you can decide what material to choose.

Clothing materials

The clothing materials which are usually available in Africa are cotton, linen, silk, rayon, wool, synthetic, or man-made, materials and mixtures of these.

Cotton grows in most parts of Africa and the tropics. A substantial amount of the cotton used in textile factories is grown in the same country. This is especially true of Nigeria and East Africa. Cotton materials are cool, hard-wearing, easy to wash and are probably the most suitable materials for our warm weather.

Linen is produced from the bark of certain trees. It is not produced in Africa but is imported which makes it rather expensive. Linen materials are usually heavier than cotton ones, but they are cool. They also wear well and are easy to wash.

Silk comes from a caterpillar known as a silk worm. It is produced mainly in Asia and the Far East and is imported into African countries. Silk materials are very expensive. They do not withstand frequent hand-washing and are not as hard-wearing as cotton or linen. However, they are cool, light, and suitable for the tropics.

Rayon is sometimes referred to as artificial silk. It is made from wood pulp and is imported into Africa. Rayon materials are cool and light. They wash easily, but are not as hard-wearing as cotton or linen.

Wool is made from the coat of temperate breeds of sheep and is imported into Africa. Tropical sheep are more suitable for food and leather production. Woollen materials are very warm and are generally not suitable for tropical climates, except in particularly cool weather. They are hard-wearing but tend to shrink with ordinary hand-washing.

Synthetic or man-made materials are made from petroleum products and are imported from those countries which have petrochemical industries. Apart from cotton materials, they are the most easily available dress materials in African countries. There are different types of synthetic material, the most common ones being nylon and polyester. Some synthetic materials are cheap, others are expensive. Nylon materials tend to be too warm especially in hot weather. Lightweight polyester is cooler and is more hard-wearing than nylon. Both materials wash well and may not require ironing. However, both tend to collect static electricity during the harmattan. Some synthetic materials irritate the skin, some are inflammable, while others cannot be hand-washed and have to be dry-cleaned. These types are therefore not suitable for making clothes, particularly for infants.

Cotton and wool fibres are sometimes mixed with one another, or with other fibres, to produce different types of dress material. Many imported clothes for infants are made from these mixed materials. The label attached to the item of clothing will usually state the composition of the material used and also whether it should be hand-washed or dry-cleaned.

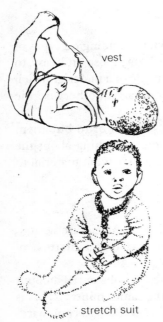

vest

stretch suit

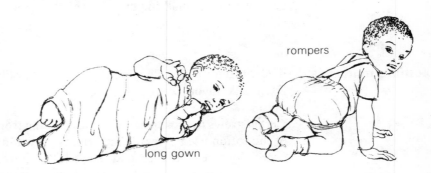

rompers

long gown

Ready-made infant clothing

Various types of ready-made infant clothing are available in the markets. Some are imported while others are made locally. The main types are mentioned here.

Vests	These are usually made from cotton, synthetic or mixed material and are available in different sizes. Some have sleeves, others do not. Some have round necks while others wrap around the infant and are tied with tapes. The advantage of the latter type is that the vest does not have to be pulled over the baby's head, which some babies dislike. Vests are used mainly as undergarments for cool weather but may also be used as sole garments on a hot day.
Pants	These come in various sizes and are usually made from nylon or other man-made materials. Some are lined with a light, plastic, waterproof material. Pants vary widely in quality and price. The pretty frilly ones are attractive but they are usually made of fine nylon and do not last long. When buying a pair of pants, remember that they have to be worn *over a nappy* so you must allow enough room.
Long gowns	These are made from various materials and may have long or short sleeves. They are useful for day- or night-wear for newborn babies and infants under six months old but are not suitable as day-wear for infants older than six months. This is because most infants begin to crawl at this stage and long gowns would restrict the movement of their legs.
Rompers	These are ideal for infants who have started to crawl or walk. They allow free movement of the legs and are suitable for both boys and girls. Traditionally, however, they are worn mainly by boys.
Stretch suits	These are one-piece suits which cover the whole body and either have long zips or buttons. They are made from stretch material and can be worn either during the day or at night. However, they are usually too warm for day-wear in tropical countries except during cool weather. They are perhaps most useful for really cold nights. If you do decide to buy a stretch suit remember again to buy one with enough room to allow for the nappy.
Dresses and two-piece suits	There are plenty of these on the market. They come in different shapes and styles. The materials used vary widely but are usually cotton or man-made fibres. The sizes also vary widely from tiny sizes for newborn babies to larger sizes for infants of various ages. Some of the dresses have matching pants. Traditionally, dresses are for girls and suits for boys, however, some of the suits can equally well be worn by girls.
Knitwear	Knitwear is mainly imported although an increasing number of African women now knit both for home use and for commercial purposes. Dresses, two-piece suits, pullovers, cardigans, jumpers, socks, mittens and caps can all be knitted using wool mixtures, nylon and other synthetic fibres. Like stretch suits, knitwear, in whatever shape or form, is usually too warm for a tropical climate and is worn only in really cold weather.
Pyjamas	Pyjamas for toddlers are sometimes available in the markets. They are useful as night-wear but tend to be expensive. It is much cheaper to make them yourself.
Traditional clothes	Traditional clothes vary from one area to another. Generally, they consist of a loose top and trousers for boys or a wrapper for girls. Occasionally,

small sizes suitable for toddlers are available in markets but more often they are made at home or by the family tailor.

A complete suit could be worn by a toddler but the top alone is more manageable and suitable as everyday wear, particularly when the weather is warm.

Nappies

Nappies are used mainly by mothers in urban areas who can afford them but it is hoped that the use of nappies will steadily increase over the years as incomes rise.

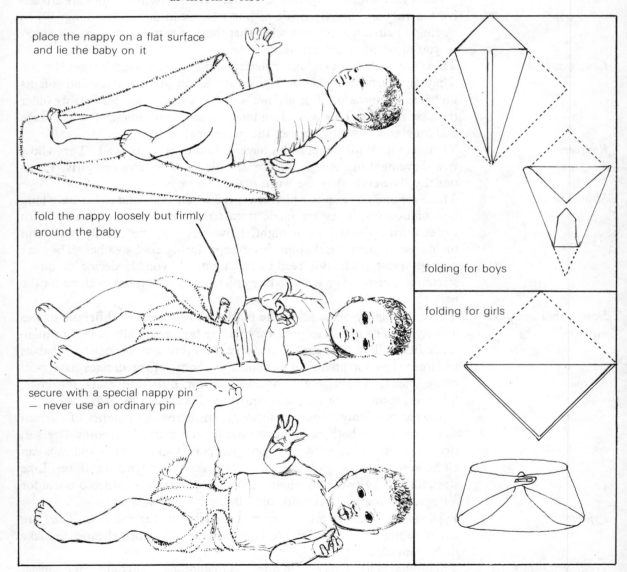

place the nappy on a flat surface and lie the baby on it

fold the nappy loosely but firmly around the baby

secure with a special nappy pin — never use an ordinary pin

folding for boys

folding for girls

Fig 6.1   Folding nappies.

Nappies are made from cotton material and vary in thickness and quality. The shapes and sizes also differ, some are square, some oblong and others triangular in shape. As a rule, nappies made from the thicker materials are better and last longer than those made from lighter materials. They are more expensive but, in the long run, are more economical.

Disposable nappies, made from paper materials, are sometimes available in the larger stores. They are the least economical but are very useful for travelling purposes.

Disposable nappy liners

These are extra-strong pads made from tissue paper and are sometimes sold in large departmental stores. As the name implies, they are used to line the inside of ordinary nappies in order to protect them from excessive soiling. The liners are usually designed to keep the moisture away from the baby's body after it has been absorbed, so keeping the baby drier and more comfortable. Some mothers use ordinary paper tissues as nappy liners but the tissues tend to disintegrate easily when they become wet and are therefore not very effective.

Washing nappies

Nappies are made from white cotton material and tend to turn greyish in colour if not properly washed. In any case, nappies must always be washed very thoroughly for hygienic reasons. To keep your baby's nappies fresh, white and clean you must first rinse the soiled nappy thoroughly to remove as much of the baby's waste as possible and then soak the nappy for one or two hours in water, or sterilising solution, containing soap powder or detergent. (If you bottle-feed your baby, the sterilising solution which you used for sterilising the bottle on the previous day may come in useful here.) Finally, wash and rinse the nappy thoroughly to remove all traces of detergent (see colour plate 3).

It is not advisable to use bleach because this can cause rashes.

Clothing for warm weather

Clothing for newborn babies has already been discussed in Chapter 2 and general guidelines for clothing infants were discussed at the beginning of this chapter.

A young baby's ability to regulate his body temperature is not as effective as that of older children or adults. He will tend to lose heat rather than conserve it.

In warm weather, infants require very little clothing. One layer of light clothing over a nappy and a pair of pants is more than adequate. Short sleeves are preferable to long sleeves (see colour plate 4).

Clothing for cool weather

Two layers of clothing are usually adequate for cool weather particularly when the clothes are made of a warm material such as flannel. Vests are useful as undergarments. For really cold weather, as sometimes occurs at night during the harmattan season, a third layer of clothing may be necessary. This is where knitted pullovers and cardigans are useful (see colour plate 4).

Night-wear

The practice of allowing infants to sleep in the clothes which they have been wearing during the day is not at all hygienic for obvious reasons. Unfortunately, this practice is common.

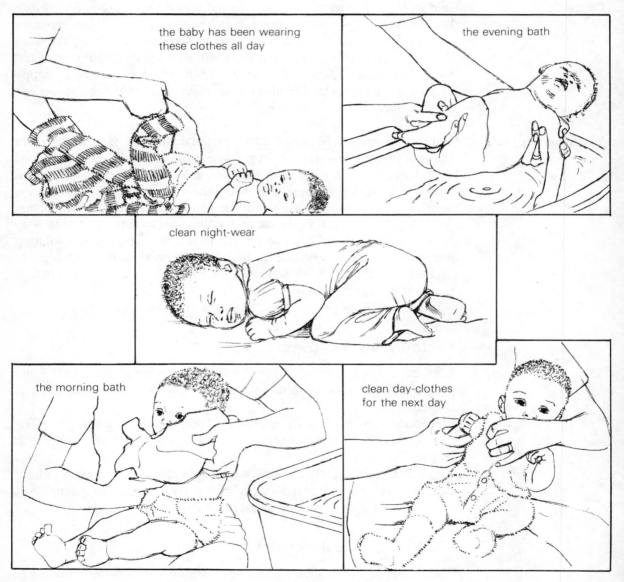

Fig 6.2   The baby should have separate night- and day-wear.

54

After his evening bath (see colour plate 2), the infant's clothes should be changed. Ordinary long gowns are quite adequate as night-dresses for young infants of both sexes. Infants of approximately one year of age or more should be provided with pyjamas (for boys) and proper night-dresses (for girls), although girls may equally well wear pyjamas. Night-dresses are almost the same as long gowns except that they are often made from prettier material.

After his bath the following morning, change his night-clothes for fresh, clean day-clothes. It is unhealthy to dress infants in the clothes which they wore on the previous day as these clothes will invariably be soiled with sweat, dirt and dust (see Fig 6.2).

Nutrition

The purpose of nutrition

The purpose of nutrition is to provide the body with the energy and materials needed for the growth and maintenance of body tissues. The tissues of the body are constantly changing; old or worn out tissues are replaced by new ones. Children who are still growing are constantly laying down more bone, muscle and other tissues.

For work, play and the maintenance of health the body requires the nutrients provided by food (see pages 57-60). Water is not always called a nutrient but it is essential for our body fluids and, as everyone knows, is vital to life. Drinking enough water and preventing excessive loss of water from the body are as important to good health as is the correct diet.

The nutritional value of food

In order to be able to prepare a balanced and nutritious diet, it is important for us to know the nutritional value of our common foods.

Meat

In African countries meat is obtained mainly from cows, goats, sheep, pigs and poultry. Meat from all these animals has approximately the same nutritional value.

Meat is an important source of high quality protein and fat. It contains vitamin B and minerals, particularly iron. Liver is also rich in vitamins A and D.

Fish

A large variety of fish is available in this country. Fish has roughly the same nutritional value as meat but it contains less iron. The soft, edible fish bones are a good source of calcium. Fish livers are very rich in vitamin D. Crayfish, lobsters and crabs have the same food value as fish.

Eggs

These are good sources of high quality protein and fat. Protein is present in the white of the egg while fat is present mainly in the yolk.

Eggs are also rich in minerals and vitamins, especially calcium and vitamins A and D.

Milk and milk products

The high nutritional value of milk has already been emphasised in an earlier chapter. Milk is a good source of calcium and vitamin D for growing children but it is a poor source of iron.

Nutritional requirements

To carry out its various functions the body needs carbohydrates, fats, protein, minerals and vitamins.

Carbohydrates

Foods rich in carbohydrates come mainly from vegetable sources. Some of the more common sources of carbohydrates are cassava, cocoyams, sweet potatoes, yams, maize, plantains, rice and potatoes.

Carbohydrate is converted into glucose by the process of digestion. The glucose is absorbed through the wall of the intestine into the bloodstream. It is then transported to every organ in the body where it is broken down to release energy for work, and heat to maintain the body's temperature. Any glucose which is not immediately required is converted into fat and stored in the body.

Sugar is also a carbohydrate.

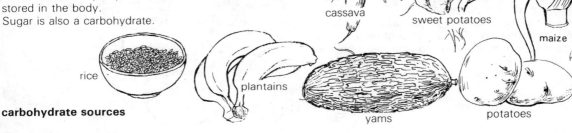

cocoyams

cassava

sweet potatoes

maize

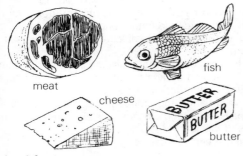

rice

plantains

yams

potatoes

carbohydrate sources

Fats

These come from both animal and vegetable sources. The main sources of animal fat available in Africa are meat, fish, butter and cheese. Vegetable fat comes mainly from oils such as palm oil, groundnut oil, and coconut oil and from margarine.

meat

fish

cheese

butter

animal fat sources

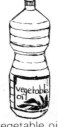

vegetable oils

margarine

vegetable fat sources

Animal fat is richer and more nutritious than vegetable fat. This is because it contains more of the essential fatty acids which cannot be manufactured by the human body and must therefore be provided in the diet.

Fat is digested and converted into fatty acids and glycerol which are then put to various uses. Like glucose, fatty acids are burned to produce heat and energy. Some are stored in certain areas of the body to be used when necessary. These areas include the layer of fat immediately beneath the skin, around the kidneys and in the spaces between certain muscle fibres.

Besides acting as an energy store, the layer of fat under the skin protects against the cold. It is well known that fat people do not feel the cold as much as thin people do. Fat-soluble vitamins can only be taken into the body with fatty foods.

African people eat mainly vegetable fat. This is not disadvantageous since it is now known that eating too much animal fat can make people prone to certain diseases of the heart and blood vessels.

Nutritional requirements

Protein

This also comes from animal and vegetable sources.
Protein is broken down in the body into amino-acids.
As in the case of essential fatty acids, there are
essential amino-acids which must be provided in the
diet. Animal protein contains more essential amino-
acids than vegetable protein does and is consequently
superior. The main sources of animal protein available
in Africa are meat, fish, crayfish, snails, eggs and
milk. Vegetable protein comes mainly from beans,
groundnuts, melon seeds, rice and green vegetables.
Protein provides the material which the body requires
for growth and repair. Every organ of the body is
made from protein. Growing children clearly require
more protein than adults, who have stopped growing,
and yet adults still require protein for the repair and
replacement of worn out tissues.

Protein foods, particularly those containing animal
protein, are expensive. The high cost of protein foods
and the failure of many people to appreciate the
importance of protein probably explains why the
average African diet often contains too little protein.

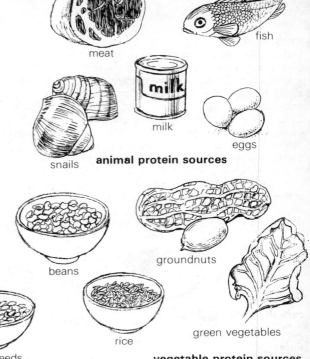

meat

fish

milk

eggs

snails

animal protein sources

beans

groundnuts

melon seeds

rice

green vegetables

vegetable protein sources

Minerals

These are present in the body mainly in the form of
salts, the most common of which are sodium,
potassium and calcium salts. Sodium and potassium
salts are widespread in nature and are particularly
plentiful in fruits and vegetables. Common table salt is
a sodium salt.

About fifty per cent of bony tissue consists of calcium
salts. The human body also contains other minerals of
which iron is the most important.

Iron is essential for the production of red blood cells.
Fish, snails, milk, eggs, beans and okra are common
sources of calcium. Meat, fish, liver, snails, melon
seeds and green vegetables are common sources of
iron.

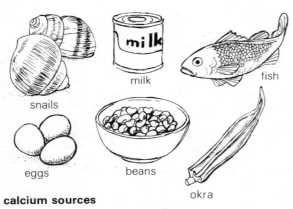

snails

milk

fish

eggs

beans

okra

calcium sources

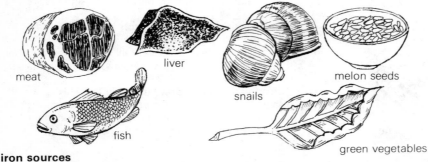

meat

liver

snails

melon seeds

fish

green vegetables

iron sources

Nutritional requirements

Vitamins

Vitamins are necessary for the health and proper functioning of the various organs of the body. They are chemical substances which are essential for life, but which the body cannot manufacture, and must therefore be provided in the diet.

Vitamin requirements vary from one animal species to another. For example, vitamin C is a vitamin needed by man but not by cows because cows can manufacture this vitamin inside their bodies.

Six vitamins which are essential to humans have now been identified. They are vitamins A, B, C, D, E and K. Human diets usually contain enough vitamin E and vitamin K but in some countries, newborn babies are given a vitamin K injection to increase the amount of vitamin K in their bodies. As far as a child's diet is concerned, the important vitamins are vitamin A, B, C and D. Some good sources of these vitamins are shown here.

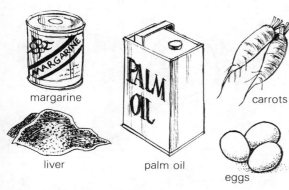

Vitamin A is important for healthy eyes and skin and for the lining of the urinary, respiratory and digestive organs. An inability to see in the dark is an early sign of vitamin A deficiency. Vitamin A is soluble in fat and so is called a fat-soluble vitamin. Common sources of vitamin A are palm oil, margarine, eggs, liver and carrots.

margarine

liver

palm oil

carrots

eggs

vitamin A sources

Vitamin B is actually a group of vitamins sometimes referred to as the vitamin B complex. This group of vitamins is required by every tissue in the human body, especially the tissues of the heart, brain and nerves. Vitamin B is also required for blood production. It is a water-soluble vitamin.

Deficiency of vitamin B causes anaemia and nervous disorders.

Common sources of vitamin B are meat, fish, yeast, groundnuts, brown bread, brown rice and mushrooms.

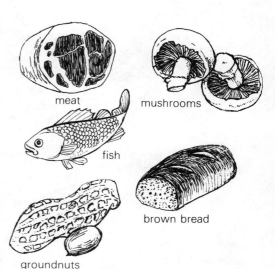

meat

mushrooms

fish

brown bread

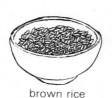

brown rice

groundnuts

vitamin B sources

Nutritional requirements

Vitamin C is another water-soluble vitamin. It is widespread in nature and is present in large amounts in fresh fruit and vegetables. Unfortunately, it is very unstable and is easily destroyed by boiling, so there is less vitamin C in cooked fruit and vegetables than in raw fruit and vegetables. Vitamin C is necessary for the health of the lining of the blood vessels. Bleeding of the gums is one of the signs of vitamin C deficiency.

Common sources of vitamin C are oranges, lemons, grapefruit, tomatoes, potatoes, plantains and green vegetables.

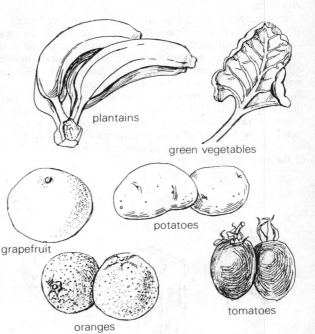

plantains

green vegetables

potatoes

grapefruit

tomatoes

vitamin C sources

lemons

oranges

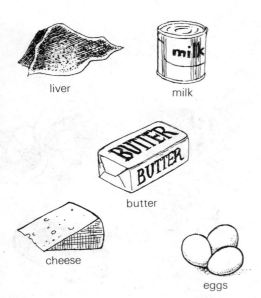

liver

milk

butter

cheese

eggs

vitamin D sources

Vitamin D is a fat-soluble vitamin and is required to strengthen all bony tissues including the teeth. Bones and teeth cannot grow in the absence of this vitamin. It is therefore a very important vitamin for growing children. Lack of vitamin D can cause stunted growth, limb deformities, hunchback and poorly developed teeth.

Common sources of vitamin D are liver, milk, eggs, butter and cheese. Vitamin D is also produced by a chemical substance which is present in the human skin. This substance is converted into vitamin D through the action of the sunlight.

Butter is made from concentrated milk fat. It is therefore a good source of animal fat as well as being a source of vitamins A and D. It is imported and is very expensive.

Cheese, which like butter is made from milk, contains not only fat but also plenty of protein. It is therefore more nutritious than butter. However, it is not a popular food item; it has to be imported and is more expensive than butter.

Root vegetables

The main root vegetables grown in Africa are cassava, yam, sweet potato, cocoyam and Irish potato. They all contain a lot of carbohydrate but have very little protein and hardly any fat. Vitamin C is the only vitamin they contain in appreciable amounts but this is largely destroyed during the process of cooking.

Cassava is the most popular of all the root vegetables. The favourite preparation of cassava is known as **gari** and is the staple food in many parts of West Africa. However, a large part of the carbohydrate or starch content is removed during the preparation of gari with the result that hardly any food value is left.

Fresh cassava contains certain poisonous salts known as cyanates. Most of the cyanates are removed during the fermentation of cassava which is a major part of the preparation of gari. Some communities eat unfermented cassava and may suffer from cyanate poisoning especially if they eat certain types of cassava.

Grains

These are also called cereals. Rice, maize, millet and sorghum (guinea corn) are the most common grains in African countries. They contain mainly carbohydrate. In addition, they contain a reasonable quantity of protein and vitamin B. They are therefore richer and more nutritious than root vegetables.

The protein and vitamin B are present mainly in the outer coat of the grain. When the outer coat is removed during processing most of these are lost. For example, white or polished rice contains less protein and vitamin B than does brown or unpolished rice.

Maize is often ground and the carbohydrate extracted. The resulting paste is used to prepare a gruel known as **pap**. This is used to feed weaning infants in many parts of Africa.

Beans

These belong to the group of vegetables known as pulses. Two types of beans are available in African countries, these are the ordinary beans and soya beans. Beans contain a lot of protein and carbohydrate. They are the main source of protein in many African homes. Soya beans contain more protein and are consequently superior to ordinary beans but they are not as pleasant tasting.

Vegetable oils

These form a significant part of an African diet. Palm oil is the most popular followed by groundnut oil. Others are coconut oil, melon seed oil and corn oil. Other vegetable oils are imported and used by a large section of the community.

Vegetable oils are the main sources of fat in the diet. They do not contain any carbohydrate, protein, vitamins or minerals. The exception to this is palm oil which is a source of vitamin A. The margarine available in African countries is made from palm oil. It is used mainly as a substitute for butter. Its nutritional value is the same as that of palm oil.

Fruit and vegetables

Fruit and vegetables are present all the year round. Green vegetables are particularly plentiful during the rainy season.

Fruit is a good source of carbohydrate, vitamin C and various salts. Citrus fruit such as oranges, grapefruit and lemons are very rich in vitamin C. The carbohydrate in fruit can be easily digested and is readily absorbed by the body. Fruit is consequently a good source of carbohydrate for small infants. Carrots, bananas, plantains, tomatoes, peppers, okra and onions also contain significant amounts of vitamin A. Carrots have a particularly high vitamin A content.

Green vegetables contain carbohydrate, vitamins and minerals including iron. The carbohydrate is cellulose fibre, which is indigestible but helps to increase bulk and prevent constipation. Some vegetables such as cassava leaves have been found to contain reasonable amounts of protein and may become useful sources of vegetable protein in the future.

Seeds and nuts

These are widely eaten all over Africa, the more popular ones being melon seeds, palm kernels, groundnuts and cashew nuts.

Seeds and nuts contain fat, in the form of oil, as well as carbohydrate, protein and some minerals. They are very useful as additional sources of protein.

Balanced diets

A person's diet is the sum total of what he eats in a day. He may eat his diet in one, two or more meals. Most African families eat an average of two meals a day.

A balanced diet is one that contains the correct proportions of carbohydrate, fat, protein, vitamins and minerals. The average diet in African countries contains mainly carbohydrate and vegetable fat and does not contain enough protein, vitamins or iron. The protein in the diet is usually vegetable protein.

A balanced diet does not have to be expensive. Animal protein can be obtained from relatively cheap sources such as iced fish, crayfish and the cheaper cuts of meat. Cereals, fruits and vegetables will supply most of the vitamin and mineral requirements. They are available throughout the year and are not too expensive.

You should ensure that your children eat some animal protein, cereals, fruit and vegetables at least once a day.

The following tables should give you some guidance as to how to feed your family a balanced diet.

	Suggested daily intake	Nutrients
Milk, cheese	¼ - ½ litre of milk 50g cheese	Protein, fat, calcium, carbohydrate, vitamin A.
Meat, fish, eggs, pulses, nuts	Two servings	Protein, fat, iron, carbohydrate, calcium, vitamins A, B and D.
Fruit and vegetables	Two servings	Vitamin C, iron, carbohydrate, calcium.
Cereals, bread, flour, rice	As required	Protein, carbohydrate, iron, vitamin B.
Fats	25g or more	Vitamins A and D.

Fig 7.1   Daily requirements of various basic foods.

Fig 7.1 shows food items grouped according to the nutrients which they contain. If, during each day's meals, something from each group has been eaten then some of all the required nutrients will have been eaten.

Breakfast	Fruit or fruit juice Vegetable dish with scrambled egg or meat stew Tea or coffee
Midday meal	Meat, vegetable or fish dish Fruit Tea or coffee
Evening meal	Soup or stew with vegetables Fruit dish Tea or coffee

Fig 7.2   Guidelines for planning a day's meals.

8   Weaning

Although breast milk is a completely adequate diet for a baby during his first six months, it becomes less so as he grows older. The iron, carbohydrate and protein contents of the breast milk gradually become inadequate for the growing child and it is therefore important that additional sources of iron, carbohydrate and protein should be added to the diet of children older than six months. By the age of six months, the infant has learned to bite and chew, showing that he is ready for foods other than milk.

Weaning is the process by which a baby's diet is changed from a milk diet to a solid or adult diet. It is a very important process in the life of all babies.

The purpose of weaning

The purpose of weaning is to provide the baby with all the nutrition he requires to grow and remain healthy. Babies grow at a faster rate during their first two years of life than at any other time in their lives. An infant doubles his birth weight by the age of five months and trebles it by the age of twelve months. By the age of two years he has grown to four times his birth weight. If the baby weighed three kilograms at birth, he would be expected to weigh six kilograms at five months, nine kilograms at twelve months and twelve kilograms at the age of two years.

Infants also require good nutrition to fight disease and stay healthy. Undernourished infants are very susceptible to all types of infection.

When he has been fully weaned, an infant should be able to eat the normal family diet. Most infants are able to do this between the ages of nine and twelve months.

General guidelines

These guidelines are meant particularly for mothers who have just had their first baby.

When to start   In medical circles, it is generally agreed that by the age of one month, an infant's digestive system is ready to cope with some types of food other than milk. However, most doctors recommend the age of three to four months as the ideal age to start weaning. However, some infants may have to start earlier.

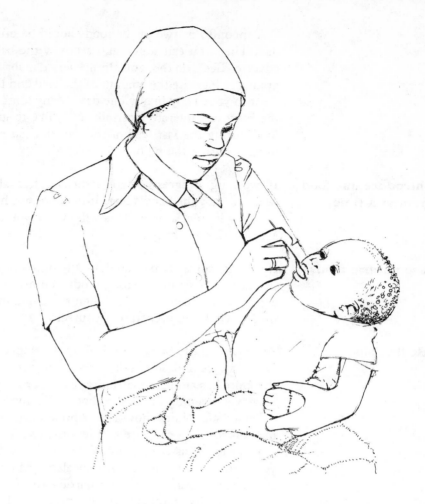

Fig 8.1
Weaning should begin
at 3-4 months.

Weaning should start well before your baby is six months old to give you enough time to introduce him to his new diet and to give him time to get used to the new foods. It should however be stressed that *milk feeds should be continued throughout the weaning process*, particularly at first when the baby can only take very small amounts of other foods.

Progress slowly

A great deal of experimentation is required during the process of weaning. Starting early gives the mother time to progress slowly.

When you are about to start weaning your baby, choose a convenient time of the day to start him off. If you do not go out to work, the middle of the morning is a good time to choose. By that time, your morning chores are over and the rest of the family are away at work or school. Another reason for choosing the mid-morning period is that you will have the rest of the day to deal with any upsets to the baby's system which may occur.

It is better to give your baby the new food before breast-feeding. If you wait until after the milk feed the new food may be refused because the baby's stomach is full.

A spoonful or two of the food should be offered once only on the first day. Then you can watch and see how the baby takes it. If there are no adverse effects do the same thing every day for about a week. You can then gradually increase the amount of the feed and the number of times you offer it to your baby in any one day. Many mothers, once they are sure that the baby can tolerate a certain food, like to give their baby his weaning food during the last feed of the day to ensure that he does not wake up hungry during the night.

Introduce one food item at a time

If weaning progresses satisfactorily, after about one month you can begin to vary the baby's diet. It is important however, that you introduce one new item at a time. This will enable you to know if any foods do not agree with your baby.

Use natural foods

If they are correctly prepared, locally purchased market food-stuffs are sufficient as a basis for weaning foods. Tinned or bottled baby food is more expensive but can be useful when travelling or when there is not enough time to cook the preparation yourself.

Be flexible

An infant's taste-buds are not fully developed and cannot distinguish between sweet and sour until about the age of six months. The mother therefore has ample opportunity to get her baby accustomed to the taste of whatever weaning foods she chooses for him.

Babies sometimes show a clear preference for one particular food. They may do so when they are still less than six months old.

You should, as far as possible, respect your baby's likes and dislikes but you may have to use a great deal of patience to persuade him to eat something which he does not particularly fancy.

Occasionally, mothers will attempt to solve this type of problem by force-feeding but this is a dangerous practice as will be explained shortly.

Fig 8.2 Suitable utensils for weaning.

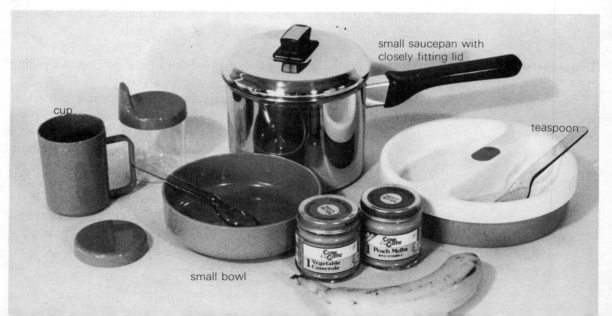

Observe strict hygiene

The need for observing strict hygiene in food preparation has been discussed in an earlier chapter. This need is even greater in the case of young infants who have little or no resistance to infection.

You should keep your baby's feeding utensils separate from those used by the rest of the family. If possible, this should also apply to the utensils you use for preparing the baby's meals. This will make it easier for you to keep them clean and free from contamination. A small saucepan with a closely fitting lid is usually sufficient for preparing the weaning foods. For crockery, a small bowl, a cup and a teaspoon are the only necessary items.

The various utensils must be thoroughly cleaned but do not have to be sterilised. All they require is to be washed thoroughly in clean water immediately after use. The bowl, cup and spoon can be kept together inside a larger bowl or container which should have a closely fitting lid.

Weaning diets

Weaning diets must be balanced diets and should contain protein, fat, carbohydrate, vitamins and minerals.

Pap

This is the most popular weaning food in African countries. It is cooked simply by adding boiling water to a paste, which is usually made from maize, and contains only carbohydrate. Pap alone is therefore very far from being a balanced diet. In order to make it more nutritious it should be enriched with either powdered milk, egg yolk, groundnut paste or crayfish powder.

Powdered milk is preferable to evaporated milk because it is cheaper and keeps better. Two scoops of the powder are enough for a cup of pap. Mix the powder with a small amount of boiled water. The mixture can then be added before or after cooking the pap.

If you prefer to use egg yolk, add it to the cooked pap and mix thoroughly. Then boil the mixture for a few minutes so that the yolk is partially cooked.

To make groundnut paste, roast fresh groundnuts until they are crisp. If you buy roasted groundnuts be careful to buy those with the skin on as it acts as a barrier against contamination and you can easily remove it yourself. Grind the roasted nuts into a fine paste. This paste will keep for several days even if it is not kept in a refrigerator. Use one teaspoon of paste for each cup of pap. The paste can be added either before or after the pap is cooked.

Crayfish powder is prepared in the same way as groundnut paste. The only difference is that the crayfish will already have been roasted. After grinding, pass the powder through a fine sieve to remove the larger particles. Keep the powder in a container with a tightly fitting lid or cover. One spoonful of the powder is enough to enrich one cup of pap. Add the powder before cooking the pap to ensure that any micro-organisms which may be present are destroyed during the process of cooking.

Brown pap is made from sorghum (guinea corn) and contains some protein and minerals. It is richer than ordinary white pap but is not as widely produced. To ensure that it meets with all the infant's requirements it should be enriched in the same way as ordinary pap.

Other grain preparations

Preparations of grains other than maize and sorghum, can be used as alternative weaning foods.

Rice flour is made locally from white or polished rice and is sold in the markets. It is relatively cheap and is quite suitable as a weaning food. It takes a little longer to cook than pap and should be enriched in the same way as pap.

Semolina is another suitable weaning food. It is produced from wheat and is sold in the market. It is also reasonably cheap and mixes best with milk. Like rice flour it takes longer to cook than pap. It is important to note that Semovita, a product related to semolina, is *not suitable for weaning*. It is made from wheat husks, is cheaper than semolina, and contains more protein and vitamins but unfortunately, it is too heavy for the digestive system of young infants.

Custard is another wheat product. Its yellow colouring is artificial. It is a suitable weaning food but is rather more expensive than pap, rice flour or semolina. There are African as well as imported brands. Custard mixes well with milk or egg yolk, the mixture being prepared in the same way as for pap.

Imported baby cereals are also made from wheat and contain added milk and vitamins. However, they are rather expensive.

Whatever weaning diet you choose should *always* be given to your baby using a cup and a small spoon. *The practice of using a feeding bottle with a large hole in the teat is not advisable.* This is because the aim is not only to teach the infant to eat an adult diet but also to teach him to eat it in an adult fashion. As many mothers have discovered, weaning a child from a bottle may prove more than a little difficult!

Changes in diet

A single weaning food is adequate during the first month of weaning. By the end of that period, the infant should be four to five months old.

At four to five months

Between the ages of four and five months, a little variety can be introduced into an infant's diet. The liquid or broth from boiled meat or fish is rich in protein, vitamins and minerals. This broth is very suitable as an additional source of these essential nutrients. It is probably cheaper and more convenient to remove some of the broth when preparing the family's soup and use this. You can reinforce the vitamin and mineral content of the broth by adding a small amount of well-cooked and finely-sieved vegetable. Spinach is ideal for this.

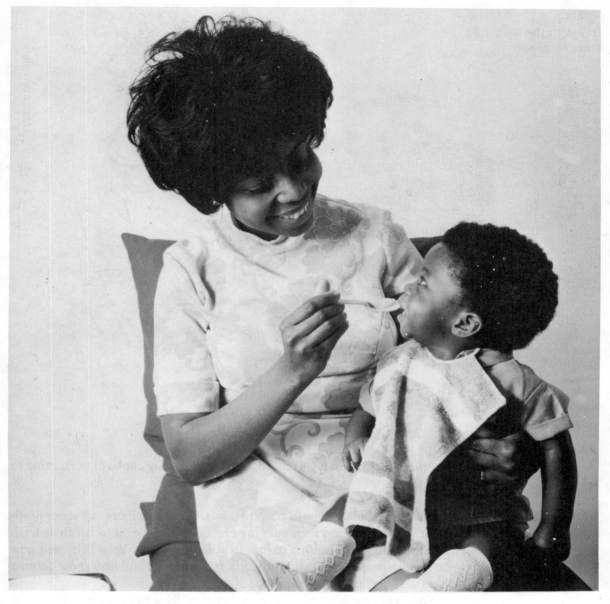

Fig 8.3   Using a cup and spoon for weaning.

At five to six months

The infant learns to hold objects at this stage and will usually try to put them into his mouth. He has already learned to bite with his gums but has not yet learned to chew. This is, nevertheless, a good time to introduce him to solid food but you must be careful to give him only food which dissolves easily in the mouth. Biscuits and pieces of bread are suitable. *Never leave the baby alone when you have given him a piece of solid food.* This is because the baby may bite off a large piece and attempt to swallow it whole since he has not yet learned how to chew. If this happens, remove

Fig 8.4
Stay with the baby
when he is eating.

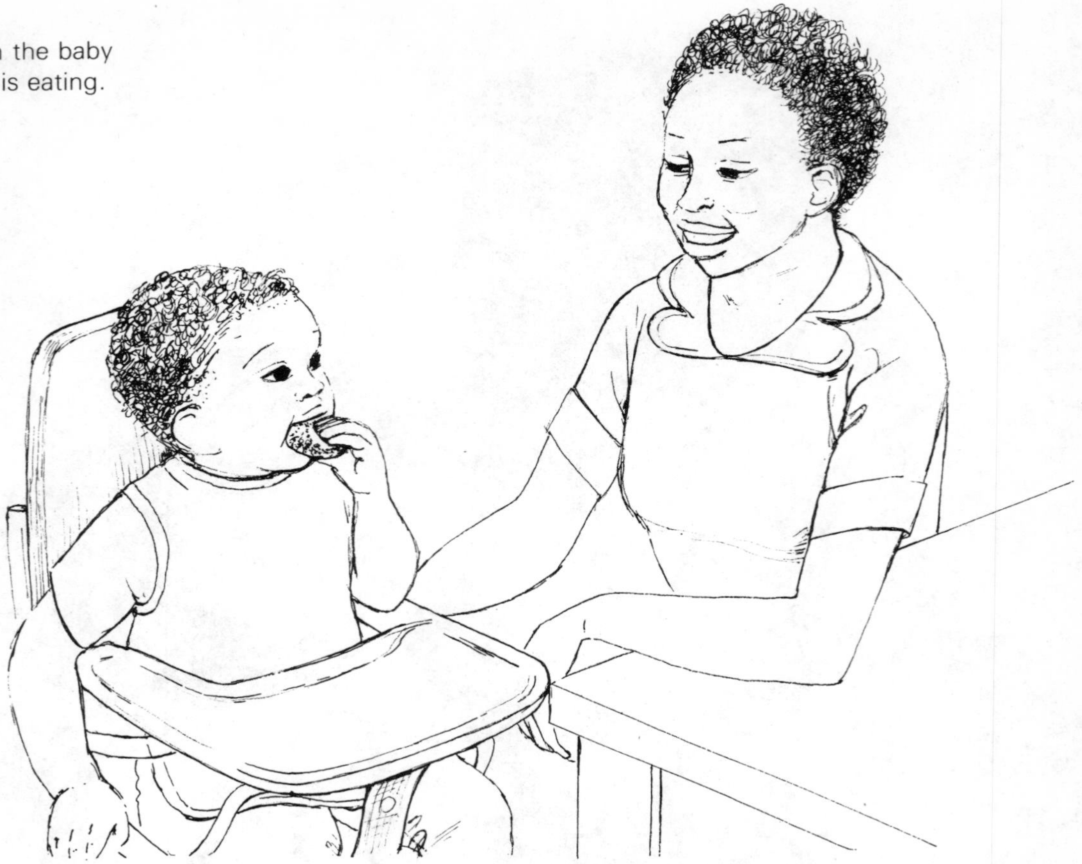

the piece from the baby's mouth, otherwise he may choke in attempting to swallow it.

At six to nine months

From the age of six months onwards, infants become more and more proficient at handling and manipulating objects. Many begin to cut their teeth and show signs of wanting to join in at family meals. Your baby will now be ready to experiment with different types of food and may show definite likes and dislikes for certain foods.

You may now offer him different types of food but always in a mashed or semi-liquid form. For example, mashed yam, potatoes, beans or very softly boiled rice would be suitable at this stage. Your baby should now be able to eat the family soup but will not be able to cope with pieces of meat. Fish, being softer, will be more acceptable to him.

The aim is to introduce him to the family diet gradually so that he will eventually be able to eat with the rest of the family.

At ten to twelve months

Weaning should be completed during this period, with the infant now able to eat the family diet without any need for modification. He still has to be fed separately and allowed plenty of time. Some mothers find it convenient

70

to feed their baby before the rest of the family. This is ideal where the mother does not go out to work and has time to finish preparing the family meal well before the family is ready for it.

As they approach their first birthday, many infants begin to show signs of wanting to feed themselves. This should not be confused with the desire to play with food which all infants have as soon as they are old enough to play. If your baby shows signs of wanting to feed himself you should teach and encourage him.

After twelve months

Until your baby is well over two years old, he should not be allowed to eat from the same bowl as that used by his older sisters and brothers. He may have a large appetite but cannot eat at the same speed as his elders and so may only be able to eat a very small share of the family meal. It is important to remember that as soon as he starts to crawl your baby will use much more energy and so need a large amount of food in proportion to his size.

Introducing particular foods

Fruit

Fruit is a ready source of carbohydrate, minerals and vitamins and is very useful as an additional source of energy.

From the age of one month, an infant can take fruit juices quite comfortably. He will be ready for whole fruit as soon as he can grasp and hold on to objects. You should make it a practice to give your baby fruit or fruit juice at least once a day as soon as he can take them.

Fig 8.5   A baby will be ready for fruit as soon as he can grasp.

Fig 8.6   You should give your baby fruit juice as part of his weaning diet.

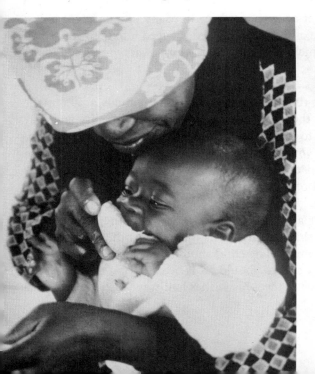

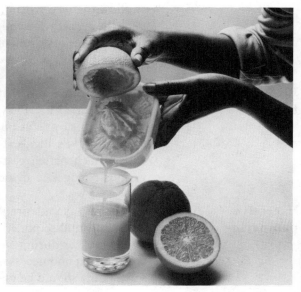

71

Vegetables

Vegetables are more difficult to digest than fruit but are useful sources of minerals, vitamins and sometimes protein. They are often used for seasoning in the preparation of soup dishes and are well cooked in the process. This helps to soften the fibres and so make them more digestible. Infants who cannot yet digest vegetables usually pass them out unaltered in the stool. If this happens it is better to take vegetables out of the weaning diet for a couple of weeks.

Vitamin supplements

In cold countries, where the rays of the sun are weak for most of the year, only small amounts of vitamin D are produced by the action of sunlight on the skin. In addition, fruit and vegetables do not grow and may become scarce during the winter months. Infants in these countries may need extra supplements of some vitamins in addition to those which they gain from their diet.

In tropical countries, where the rays of the sun are always strong and fruit and vegetables are available throughout the year, vitamin supplements should not be necessary provided the infant is fed adequately with a balanced diet. However, if you are worried that your baby is not getting an adequate, balanced diet many brands of vitamin preparations are sold in the chemists' shops and most of them are reasonably cheap.

Weaning problems

Weaning should be a gradual and flexible process but you must remember that there are some things you should not do while weaning your baby.

Force-feeding

This is a dangerous practice but unfortunately still takes place. The nostrils of the infant are covered with the back of the hand while the palm is used to pour the feed into his mouth. As a result, the infant is forced to swallow the feed whenever he gasps for breath. Many infants have choked to death in this way while others have inhaled the feed into their lungs and so have developed pneumonia. *Force-feeding has no advantages at all and must never take place.*

Fighting with the baby

Infants become aware of themselves as separate individuals at about the age of six months. They then begin to assert their individuality and may try to do this by refusing to co-operate at mealtimes. You will only play into your child's hands if you allow yourself to be drawn into a battle of wills. Much patience and understanding is required in dealing with the various changes in mood of a growing infant.

Excessive pampering

This is just as undesirable as fighting with your baby. In the case of many spoilt and undisciplined children, the basis for their conduct is often laid by the mother during weaning. The child should be made to realise that it is important and necessary that he should do as he is told. At the same time some effort should be made to meet his wishes half-way. There are no hard and fast rules as to how you may achieve this happy medium. Each case has to be handled on an individual basis, with the infant and his mother both learning as they progress.

Overfeeding

It is now known that obesity in later life can be caused during infancy by feeding babies with too many sugary foods. Although it is important that an infant should be well fed it is equally important that he should not be overfed.

Breast-feeding

Many mothers are tempted to stop breast-feeding when their babies have been successfully weaned but this would be a mistake. Apart from the high food value of breast milk, the protective antibodies in breast milk will continue to be needed by the infant after weaning.

9 Growth and development

Growth simply means an increase in size. Development, on the other hand, is more complex and involves an increasing ability to perform various skills, whether physical or intellectual.

Growth and development take place simultaneously in a child. Both processes affect one another and cannot be separated but, by closely observing growing children, doctors have come to realise that there are several forms of growth and development and that these occur simultaneously.

Physical growth

This begins the moment the child is conceived in the womb, and continues until the child reaches adulthood. It involves the building of new tissues as well as the increasing in size of individual existing tissues. As the child grows, he increases in height and weight.

Physical growth also involves changes in the shape of the body. The shape of a newborn infant is not the same as that of a two-year-old and both have a different body shape from that of an adult. The various changes in body shape of a growing child are shown on pages 79-82.

As was mentioned earlier, tissues are built from protein. Physical growth therefore requires a continuous and adequate supply of good quality protein food.

Mental development

The main difference between man and other animals is that certain parts of the human brain are more highly developed with the result that man possesses a more highly developed intellect.

During pregnancy and the first two years of life, the child's brain grows at a faster rate than the rest of his body. To allow the brain to undergo this rapid growth, the bones of the skull of an infant are only loosely joined together. There are four pairs of skull bones, one of each pair being on the right and the other on the left side of the head. Where more than three bones meet, a space is left which forms a small depression. This space varies in size and is known as a **fontanelle**. There are six fontanelles but the two most important ones are known as the anterior and posterior fontanelles.

The anterior fontanelle is the larger of the two and is situated towards

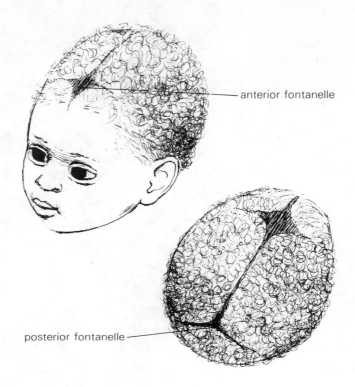

Fig 9.1
Positions of the fontanelles.

anterior fontanelle

posterior fontanelle

the front of the head in the centre. The pulse can often be seen or felt at this point. The anterior fontanelle becomes smaller as the infant grows older and disappears when the infant is between fifteen and eighteen months old.

It is not very easy to see or feel the posterior fontanelle. It is situated near the middle of the back of the head and is smaller than the anterior fontanelle. It disappears by the time the infant is three months old.

Unless a child's brain is healthy his intellect cannot develop and the child will not be able to learn. Education helps the child to learn but only if the brain is healthy.

Emotional development

Fear, anger, hate, joy and love are all human emotions. A growing child must learn to react to different situations with the appropriate emotions. When we say that a person is childish we mean that his emotional reactions are like those of a child.

A mother's love is extremely important in the emotional development of her child because love encourages a feeling of security, and when a child feels secure he will not be afraid to react appropriately to different situations. Breast-feeding promotes emotional development in the child as it is

Fig 9.2
A mother's love is
extremely important.

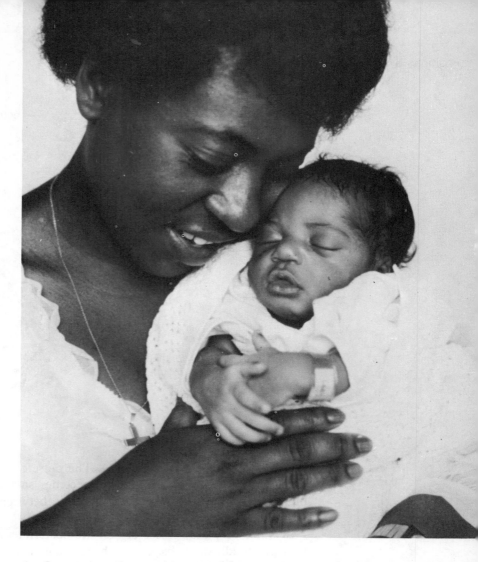

the first and earliest way in which a bond of love is established between a mother and her child.

Social development

Human beings are said to be social animals, meaning that they generally prefer not to live alone. They need the company of others to be contented and happy. As part of a child's development, he must learn how to behave in order to be acceptable to the other members of the community. A child makes his first social contact when he smiles at his mother which happens when he is about six weeks old.

Doctors are becoming increasingly aware of the importance of proper social development, a lack of which can result in delinquency. Delinquent children are known by their antisocial behaviour which may include stealing, lying or even violence.

Influencing factors

Growth and development are greatly affected both by heredity and by the environment in which the child is growing.

We can do nothing to change our heredity, but we can do a fair amount to influence our environment. The environmental factors which are most important to the development of children are nutrition, hygiene, parental love and the discipline imposed on them by their parents. These factors are discussed here.

Heredity

Heredity is determined by simple chemical substances known as **genes**. There are thousands of genes in the human body, working in pairs. A child receives one half of each pair of his genes from his mother and the other half from his father. Each pair of genes has a special function. The colour of our skin, our adult height and so on are all determined by the type of genes we possess.

Genes are greatly influenced by the environment. For example, if a child has genes which suggest that he will be tall, he will not reach his full stature unless he is provided with enough protein food. If he lives in a poor home environment where food is scarce, he will not become as tall as his genes indicated.

Nutrition

The importance of good nutrition, especially in infancy, has already been stressed. A child will not grow well unless he is well fed. Genes require materials with which to work and build, and these are supplied mainly by the food we eat. For example, even if your child has genes for keen eyesight, his vision will be poor unless enough vitamin A is supplied in his diet. Similarly, if an architect has planned a beautiful house, it will not achieve that beauty if the builder uses poor materials.

Good nutrition also helps to prevent and fight infection which invariably retards growth and development.

Hygiene

Good hygiene is very important. Some children do not grow well because they live in unhygienic surroundings and so suffer from severe and repeated infections. As many experienced mothers know, a young child who has learned to walk before being attacked by a severe illness such as measles may stop walking as a result of the illness and then have to learn to walk all over again.

Parental love

A mother's love is important in the emotional development of her child, particularly during the first two years of the child's life. Infants who are deprived of their mother's love tend to become nervous and insecure adults.

It should be pointed out that the mother's love need not come from the biological or natural mother. She could be a foster mother. It is always better to bring up a motherless child in a foster home rather than in an institu-

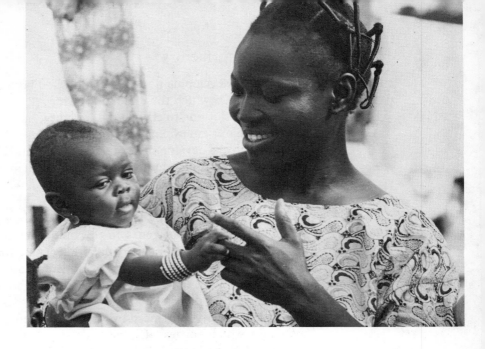

Fig 9.3
There is no substitute
for a mother's love.

tion. This is because no matter how caring the workers in the institution may be, there is no substitute for a mother's love.

Discipline

Discipline is very necessary for the social development of the child. By the time he reaches school age, the child is expected to be able to distinguish good behaviour from bad behaviour. It is therefore the parents who have the responsibility of teaching their children how to behave properly. Children who grow up without parental discipline either from their own parents or from foster parents tend not to develop socially and so find it difficult to fit into their community.

Discipline will be discussed in greater detail in the next chapter.

Fig 9.4
A baby learns to grasp
objects when he is only
a few months old.

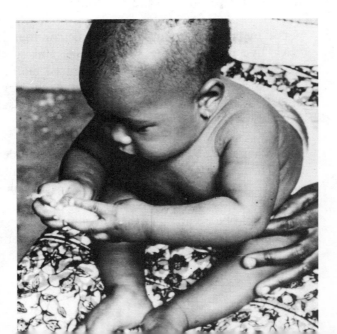

78

Growth and development at various ages

The rate at which children grow varies from child to child. It is important for mothers to realise this in order to save themselves from unnecessary anxiety. However, there is a range within which a normal child is expected to grow and develop. For example, no matter how slow the baby is, he should be able to sit by the age of nine months, stand by the age of twelve months and should be walking by the age of fifteen months or, at most, eighteen months.
This account refers to the average child. Your baby may be faster or slower.

At birth

The infant should weigh at least 2500 grams and his head should measure at least 33 centimetres at the greatest circumference.
A newborn baby assumes a folded up position which is similar to the position he assumed while in the womb. The baby cannot control his head which wobbles from side to side and his fists are held tightly clenched. The baby sleeps most of the time and expresses his needs by means of a lusty cry. The infant can be easily startled when awake, causing his whole body to tremble.
He can suck and swallow, can see large objects, can hear and smell but has no sense of taste. He has strongly developed instincts, very much like those of an animal and reacts instinctively to his mother's warmth and love.

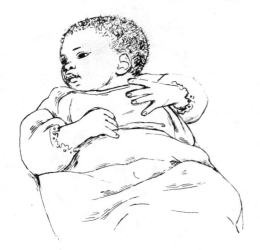

At one month

The baby begins to notice his surroundings and sleeps less often. While in his mother's arms, he fixes his gaze on her face and appears to be studying her. His head is now less wobbly, his fists are less tightly clenched and the baby is less easily startled. When he is laid face downwards on a bed, the baby can now lift his head from the bed for a brief moment.

At two months

The baby has learned to smile and to make throaty noises. He smiles at his mother whenever she talks to him. When supported in a sitting position, the baby can hold his head reasonably well although it still wobbles a little.
The infant may have started to suck his fingers. Babies start to suck their fingers by chance but they persist in doing it because it gives them a feeling of satisfaction.

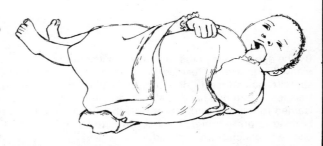

Growth and development at various ages

At three months

The baby's back and neck muscles are stronger now, he holds his head up without any wobbling and he can sit with a fairly straight back if properly supported with pillows. When laid face downwards, the baby can now lift his head and shoulders from the ground. At this stage, his fists are no longer clenched, and his hands are open. The baby cannot reach for an object but can grasp an object when it is placed in his hands.

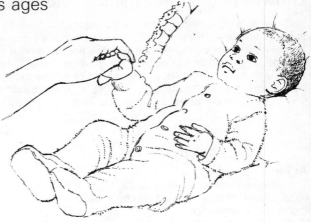

The baby takes more notice of the people around him but cannot distinguish one person from another. He is quite content to be carried by strangers.
A single weaning diet could be gradually introduced at this age over a period of about one month.

At six months

Weaning

The baby can now chew regardless of whether he has started to cut his first milk teeth. The sense of taste is now more developed and the baby should now be able to distinguish between sweet and sour tastes. Between four and five months old is a good time to start varying the baby's diet, possibly with a little broth from boiled meat or soup. Biscuits or small pieces of bread should be introduced later, at five to six months, to help your baby learn to chew.

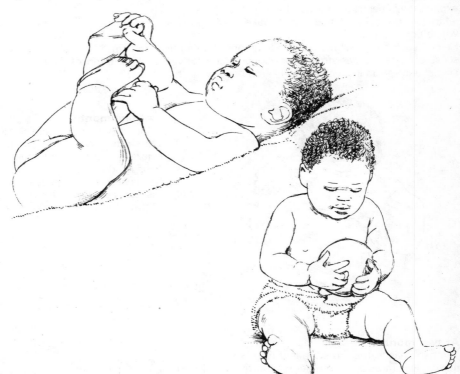

By the age of six months the baby has learned to do many things. He has learned to sit on his own without support, he can reach for an object, hold on to it, and transfer it from one hand to the other. He has also learned to roll over and may roll off the bed if there is nothing to prevent him. The baby likes to lie on his back and watch his hands and feet.

Considerable progress has been made both emotionally and socially. The baby has learned to recognise those around him and to distinguish one person from another. He prefers his mother to the rest of the family and shows definite pleasure when she approaches. The baby will show definite likes and dislikes for people and for objects such as toys.

Growth and development at various ages

At nine months

By this stage the baby should be able to crawl. He may also have started to stand
holding on to the furniture. He will be more proficient at using his hands and will
try to pick things up with his thumb and forefinger. However, the baby will find it
difficult to let go of the things he has picked up. He will still have a tendency to
put whatever he picks up into his mouth.

The ability to crawl makes it possible for the baby to
move from place to place. He shows a keen interest in
the things around him and will crawl from one part of
the room to another, exploring.

The baby's babbling noises are now more intelligible.
He can imitate familiar sounds and can pronounce
single syllables. He can understand the meaning of
certain words although he cannot say them. The baby
can also recognise his own name when he is called.

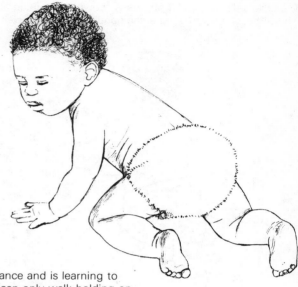

Weaning

Babies often start to cut their teeth at between six
and nine months old. Food can be varied during this
period but must always be in a mashed or semi-liquid
form. Soup is also suitable provided that the solid
pieces of food in it have been removed.

At one year

The child can now stand on his own without any assistance and is learning to
walk, or may have actually started walking. At first, he can only walk holding on
to a helping hand or to the furniture. Later, he can walk on his own without any
help. The baby begins by taking a few steps at a time.

The child's speech has also developed further. He should now be able to say two
or more words which have meaning. 'Mama' is usually the first proper word
spoken.

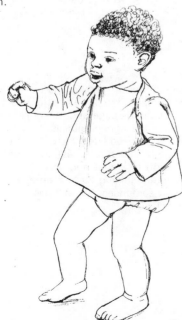

There is now less tendency for the infant to put
objects into his mouth. He can now let go of objects
and enjoys throwing things on to the floor. Any
breakable object within reach is liable to be broken.
The child can eat an adult diet, can handle a spoon
reasonably well and enjoys feeding himself.

Weaning

The child should have been gradually introduced to
the family foods so that the weaning process is
complete by the time the child is one year old. He
should now be able to eat small portions of the
normal family diet but may be fed separately, away
from the rest of the family, for convenience.

Growth and development at various ages

At fifteen months
The child can walk quite well at this stage but does so with his legs wide apart. He cannot run but can crawl upstairs using his arms and legs. He will obey simple commands but may begin to show signs of disobedience. He can help to dress himself by holding out an arm or a leg.

The child's desire to hold objects is shown by pointing at them. His ability to feed himself has improved and he can handle a cup fairly well.

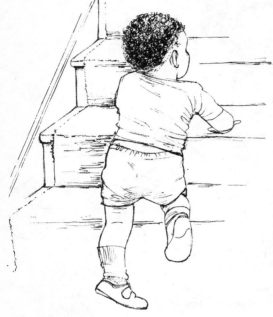

At eighteen months
The child can now walk without holding his legs wide apart; he can run for a short distance but does so rather clumsily. He can climb stairs, putting both legs on each step and can climb up and sit on a chair without assistance. The child can carry out simple orders and can name several objects.

He can say several words but mixes them together without a proper order. He should know when he is about to soil himself and should draw his mother's attention to it.

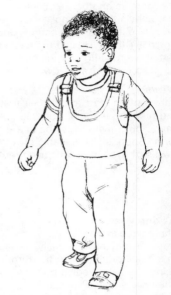

At eighteen months the child can walk.

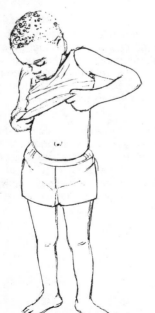

At two years
The child has become better at running and at climbing stairs. He can open doors, pull out drawers, and can open a book page by page and recognise and name pictures of some objects and animals. He can draw simple, but rather crooked lines. He can put on and take off simple clothes such as a vest and a pair of pants and can take off his shoes and socks.

The child talks incessantly, joining two or more words together to make short sentences, but still has difficulty with pronunciation.

Speech development

A child begins to say intelligible words between the ages of nine months and one year. Speech development depends on the ability to hear. A child can normally hear from the moment of birth but, if he is deaf from birth, the child will not be able to learn how to speak unless he receives special training. Speech development also depends on the degree of encouragement the child receives, in other words how often, as well as how well, his mother and others around him talk to him. The child should always be spoken to in a proper and mature manner. This is because children learn mainly by copying and if you talk to your child in childish language, he will copy your childish manner of speech. This will obviously delay the child's speech development.

Teething

There are a total of twenty milk teeth, ten in the upper jaw and ten in the lower jaw. The ten milk teeth in each jaw are divided into five identical pairs, with one of each pair on either side of the jaw. They are known by various names as shown in Fig 9.5. The four middle teeth are known as **incisors**. The teeth on either side of the incisors are known as the **canine teeth**. The two pairs of upper and lower back teeth are called **molars**.

At birth, an infant's milk teeth are already present inside the jaw. Their presence can be seen from an X-ray. However, the teeth do not start to come through until the infant is between five and seven months old.

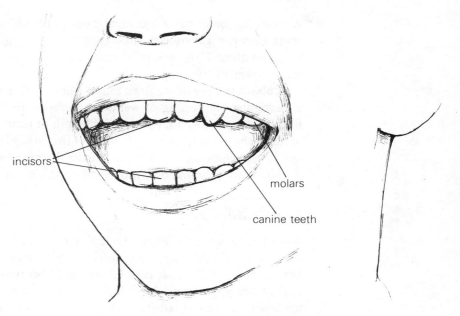

Fig 9.5 Positions of the various types of milk teeth.

There is a lot of variation in the ages at which the various teeth are cut. An infant may be born with a tooth already cut or may have none at all at the age of one year! Fig 9.6 shows the average age of cutting of the various teeth, however, your child may cut his teeth much earlier or much later than this.

Type of teeth	Average age
Central incisors	5 to 7 months
Lateral incisors	9 to 12 months
First molars	12 to 14 months
Canines	18 months
Second molars	2 years

Fig 9.6   Average age of the baby when various teeth are cut.

The teeth on the lower jaw are usually cut before the corresponding ones on the upper jaw.

Cutting teeth is usually a painless process causing, at most, a little irritability and some itching or soreness of the gums. It does *not* cause fever, diarrhoea or convulsions. It is important for mothers to note this fact. Babies still die because their illness is thought to be caused by teething with the result that they are not taken to a hospital in time.

Bladder and bowel control

A newborn baby has no control over his bladder or bowel. These two organs empty themselves automatically when they become filled with waste matter. This lack of control continues until the child enters his second year of life.

At about the age of eighteen months or a little before that, a child begins to recognise the feeling of wanting to empty his bladder or bowel but at first he is unable to hold on for any length of time. Later he learns to hold on for a short time, learning to control the bowel before the bladder. Control is better during the day than during the night when the child is asleep. Toilet training helps to improve the child's control (see Chapter 10).

Left-handedness

Most people are right-handed but about five to ten per cent of us are left-handed. During the first two years of their lives children are able to use both hands equally, that is, they are **ambidextrous**. However, as a child approaches his second birthday, he may begin to show an increasing tendency to use the left hand. It is not advisable to try and prevent left-handedness in your child, in fact it may actually be dangerous to do so.

Where nature designed the child to be left-handed, you will only make him develop emotional as well as reading and writing problems if you force him to use his right hand.

10 General care and discipline

It cannot be over-emphasised that the best person to look after a young child is his mother. Our ancestors were very aware of this fact. In traditional society a mother who had just delivered was not allowed to leave her home for a period of one month. She did not go to the market or visit her neighbours. She was excused from housework so that she could spend all her time looking after her new baby.

Fig 10.1
This method of carrying a baby is good for both mother and baby.

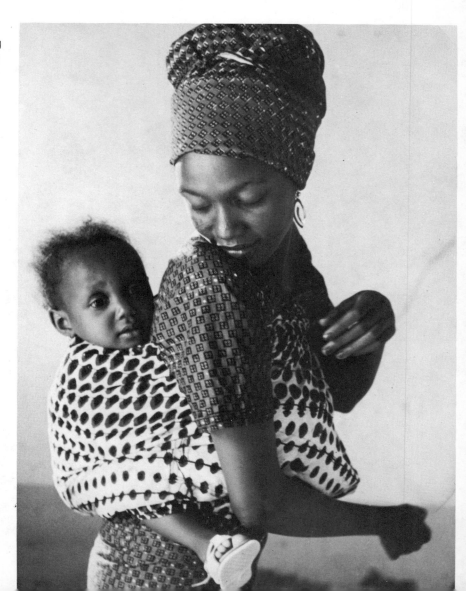

When this period of confinement was over, the new mother would go about her duties with the baby strapped to her back. In this way, she was constantly with her baby and could promptly take care of his needs. This close relationship continued until the baby stopped breast-feeding at the age of two to three years. If, for any reason, she had to leave her baby behind when she went out of the home, there were several members of the extended family unit to look after the baby in her absence.

However, things have had to be done differently in modern society. The large extended family units have tended to break up and many mothers have had to go out to work. These mothers, therefore, have to get someone to look after their baby while they are away at work.

Child-minders

A child-minder is someone who looks after a child while his mother is away from home and is usually either the baby's older sister or (occasionally) brother, a more distant relation or a hired help (usually female).

An older sister, as a rule, makes a more suitable child-minder than a more distant relation or a hired help, provided that she is not too young. She should be at least ten years old. The difficulty about this arrangement is that it interferes with the girl's schooling. Some families try to overcome this difficulty by sending the girl to an afternoon school.

A distant relation is, in turn, generally more suitable than a hired help. She should preferably be a relation of the child's mother as this makes it easier for them to get on with each other.

For obvious reasons, employing a hired help is usually the least suitable choice. Unfortunately, an increasing number of families have had to rely on this type of help. A hired help is usually a first-school leaver who, for various reasons, has been unable to proceed with her secondary education. If you have a hired help, you would be wise to give her the opportunity to further her education as you will earn her gratitude and she will co-operate more fully with you. Fortunately, there are commercial schools in most towns which operate during the afternoon or evening and would be useful in such a case.

A hired help is sometimes a middle-aged woman with no husband or children of her own to look after. This type of helper is usually difficult to find and more expensive but, being much older and more experienced than a young girl, she would be much better at looking after children.

As with many things in life, the type of hired help you end up with is very much a matter of luck. You must always remember that a child-minder is not a substitute for the child's mother and that, no matter how good your helper is, you should take over your child's care yourself as soon as you return home. You should also try to be at home as much as possible. It is unfortunate that an increasing number of mothers are leaving their young children in order to go and further their studies.

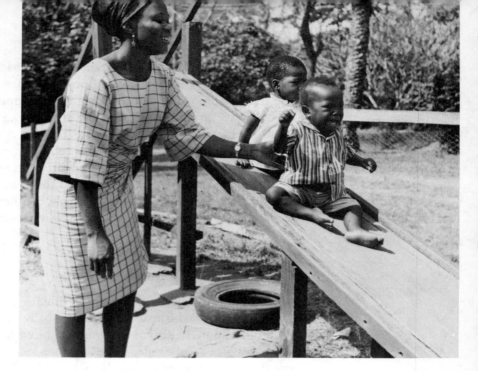

Fig 10.2
At the day-care centre.

Day-care centres

As their name implies, these are centres where young children are cared for during the day. Day-care centres were developed in industrialised countries to look after children of working mothers while they were away at work. They have recently been introduced into some African countries but are still few and far between.

Day-care centres are usually run by social organisations, although a few housewives have started to run private centres in their homes. Some centres accept babies between the ages of three months and two and a half or three years. Others accept them from a younger age. Day-care centres vary in the fee they charge but are, on the whole, very well run. In addition to general care, the children also receive useful informal education by means of toys and supervised play. They learn to get on with other children and have less difficulty in adjusting to a nursery school when their parents send them there later on.

If you have a day-care centre in your area, and the fee is reasonable, you will probably find that it is cheaper to take your child there than to employ a hired child-minder. Apart from the financial advantage, a well-run day-care centre is better for your child than a home help.

General care

Feeding, bathing and clothing infants have already been discussed but a child's care also includes protecting him against injury, providing him with facilities for play and generally helping him to develop properly.

Protection against injury

This becomes important when your baby reaches the age of three months because from that age onwards his range of movement increases quite quickly. The first thing you may discover is that your child has rolled away from where you left him. There is a danger that he may roll off his bed and injure himself, particularly if the bed is a high one. Alternatively, if he is lying on the floor in a room with an open fire he may roll over to the fire and suffer serious burns.

Your baby's range of movements will increase further when he begins to crawl. By this time he can also reach for objects and put them into his mouth. These objects may be harmful but even if they are not the child may choke while trying to swallow one of them.

When your child learns to drop things you are liable to lose your breakable possessions unless all breakable objects are kept well out of reach. As soon as your child can handle a cup he will equally be able to handle a bottle. It is natural for a child to try to eat or drink the contents of a bottle, or any container, and so you must keep dangerous drugs and poisonous liquids, such as kerosene, out of your child's reach.

The need to protect him against injury becomes more urgent when he learns to walk. Your child is then vulnerable to any danger, including that of road traffic. In addition to accidental poisoning and burns, road traffic accidents are now serious causes of injury and death in our young children.

Fig 10.3
Keep all breakable objects well out of reach.

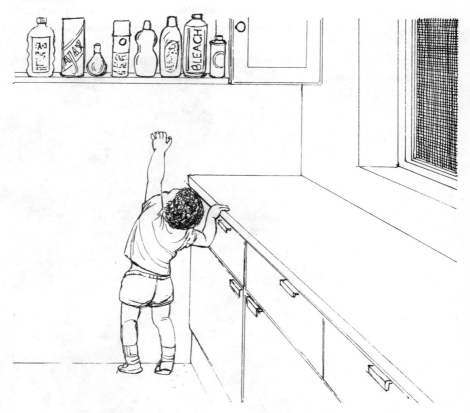

Another danger from which young children must be protected is drowning in a bath. No matter how much your child enjoys splashing in his bath, he should *never* be left alone to do so by himself.

Play facilities

Young children learn through play but this is not yet widely recognised. We tend to look on a child's play with tolerance, as something a child is allowed to do because he is too young to know better. We therefore tend not to make any special effort to provide him with facilities for playing.

Play is a form of physical and mental exercise. During play the child improves his physical and mental performance. If the child is playing with other children he is also learning how to get on with others. This helps to promote social development but, of course, there can be too much of a good thing! You should not allow your child to play at the expense of his other activities such as eating or sleeping.

Toys

Toys are an important part of a child's play. Because of the African attitude towards children's play, the importance of toys in encouraging a child's development has not yet been fully realised. Have you noticed how little girls tend to prefer dolls while the boys seem to prefer machines?

By handling and playing with toys, children learn as much as they can about the things represented by the toys. A little girl learns how to play 'mother' to her baby doll while a little boy learns all about the inside of a toy car. You can also take this as an opportunity to teach your child to value and take care of things as soon as he is old enough to learn.

Fig 10.4
Toys are an important part of a child's play.

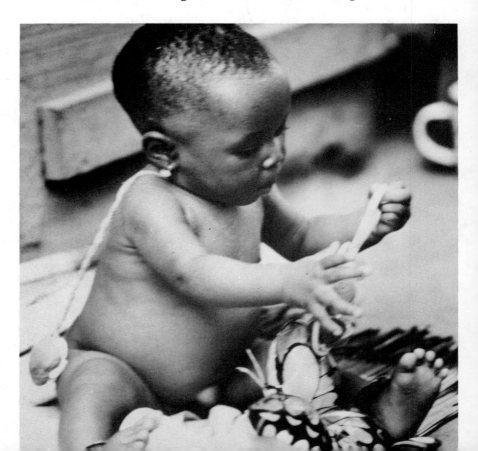

90

As soon as your child can reach for objects he is old enough to be given a toy. Toys need not be expensive but they should be made of as strong a material as possible if they are to last for a reasonable length of time! It is also important to check that the toys are safe for your baby to play with; that is, that they do not have sharp points on them or loose pieces which a child might try to swallow.

Sleeping facilities

Sleeping patterns vary as much in children as they do in adults. However, the amount of sleep a child requires decreases progressively as he grows older. A newborn baby usually needs between fifteen and eighteen hours of sleep, or even more, in a day whereas most adults need only eight to ten hours of sleep each day.

A newborn baby cannot distinguish between day and night and will sleep soundly whatever the time of day. As he grows older, he gradually learns to adjust to the sleeping hours of the rest of the family. Nevertheless, he will still need his afternoon sleep for some time to come.

Many African children sleep on mats on the floor during the night. During the day, a child may be allowed to go to sleep anywhere in the house, and quite often on the bare floor, but at night he will sleep in the same room as several other members of the family. The room may be overcrowded, which is bad for the child's health. Proper sleeping facilities should therefore be provided for young children. Ideally each child should have his own bedroom or at least a separate cot or bed. When a baby is very young his cot should be placed near his mother's bed. When the child is a little older the cot can be moved to a different part of the room or to another room altogether.

Unfortunately, separate sleeping facilities for young children are often not possible where families are large and also poor. The best that can be done in these circumstances is to see that the child does not share his bed or mat with too many people. No matter how cold the weather is, at least one window in the room should remain open to let in fresh air throughout the night.

Toilet training

It is rare to find an adult who soils himself either during the day or at night. Every child should acquire bladder and bowel control by the time he becomes an adult and most children do so before school age. However, a child can be helped to acquire control as soon as possible through toilet training.

In traditional society, a mother would feed her baby before giving him a bath. As soon as feeding had finished she would place her baby in a sitting position on her slightly parted feet. She would begin to do this when her baby had acquired control of his head at about three months. Then she

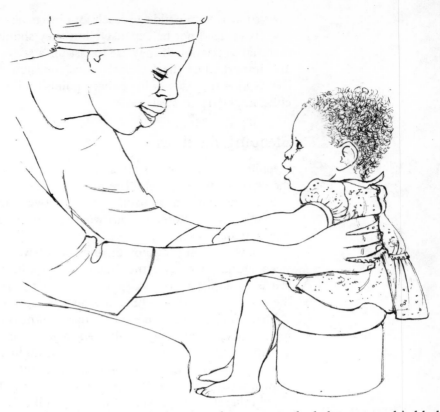

Fig 10.5
Toilet training.

would make hissing noises to try and encourage the baby to open his bladder and bowel.

Toilet training should be started as soon as the baby can sit on his own without support, which he learns to do at about the age of six months. After each of his meals you should sit the baby on a chamber pot which should be set aside for the baby's use only. He will soon learn to use the chamber pot. Later, when he starts walking, your child will go to his pot himself. At first, there will be some lapses because the child will not be able to hold on for any length of time when his bladder or bowel becomes full.

A child will acquire bowel control before bladder control. From the age of two years, a child will not normally need to wear a nappy during the day although he may continue to need one at night for some time.

Discipline

Strict discipline was rigidly maintained in traditional society. Children were supposed to be seen but not heard. A child was expected to be polite and quiet in the presence of his elders and to do only as he was told. A child would be taught strict discipline as soon as he had stopped feeding from the breast. Everybody within the family unit would take a hand in disciplining the child who would be promptly smacked whenever he did something which was considered to be wrong. This type of upbringing produced people who conformed and adhered rigidly to tradition but it also lessened their initiative and innovation.

On the other hand, modern society is now tending to go to the opposite extreme and many children grow up without enough parental discipline.

When to start

Before the age of six months, a child is not aware of himself and others around him as separate individuals. His behaviour is largely instinctive and so it is pointless to try to teach the child how to behave.

His mother is the first person a child becomes aware of as a separate individual, usually at about the age of six months. He soon realises that all his comfort comes from his mother and becomes anxious, at first subconsciously, to please her. At this point the child is ready for his mother to start disciplining him. The mother must know something about how a normal child develops, otherwise she will not know how her child should behave at various ages. For example, a six-month-old infant automatically puts an object he picks up into his mouth and should not be scolded for doing so.

How to proceed

Discipline does not only involve punishment for bad behaviour but also reward for good behaviour. Punishment and reward can both take various forms. A punishment need merely be a disapproving look or tone of voice whereas a reward can be a look of encouragement or a smile.

To be effective discipline must be applied constantly. Bad behaviour should always be punished and good behaviour always rewarded.

Fig 10.6
A typical first-aid kit for the home.

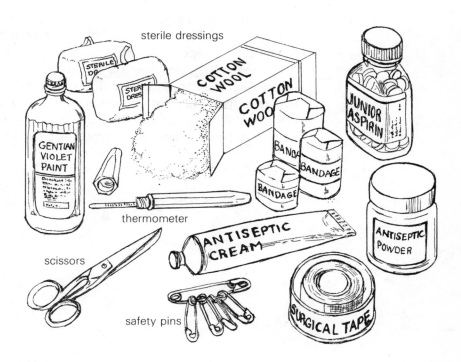

sterile dressings

thermometer

scissors

safety pins

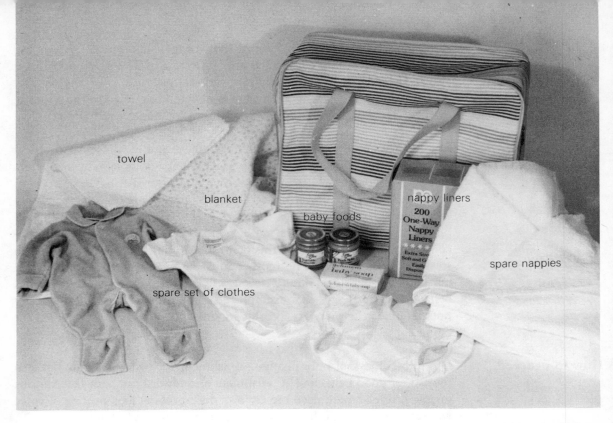

towel

blanket

baby foods

nappy liners
200
One-Way
Nappy
Liners

spare nappies

spare set of clothes

Fig 10.7 Items useful when travelling by public transport with your baby.

Discipline must always be accompanied by the good example shown by the parents. Children learn mainly by copying their parents and elders and so you cannot expect your child to behave in a certain manner if he sees you doing exactly the opposite.

It is important to remember that young children are very inquisitive, and that their incessant questioning is not a sign of forwardness or disrespect. You should therefore always try to answer your child's questions with patience and as accurately as possible.

11   Infant welfare clinics

Providing health care for any community involves three different activities. These are:
a) promoting the health of the community by the provision of good nutrition, a clean water supply and good housing,
b) preventing disease through health education, good environmental sanitation, and immunisation and
c) treating disease.

Child care is concerned with the application of these three activities to children's health. If we promote child health and do our best to prevent disease amongst our children, there will be fewer cases of disease to treat. The promotion of health and the prevention of disease are therefore more important than the treatment of disease. We should not lay too much emphasis on the treatment of disease at the expense of health promotion and the prevention of disease.

The purpose of infant welfare clinics

Infant welfare clinics are also known as child welfare clinics, well-baby clinics or simply as 'baby weighs'. In medical circles, they are frequently called under-fives clinics. The clinics look after the health of children who are less than five years old. Experience has shown that this group of children are more vulnerable to disease than older children and need extra care.

The purpose of these clinics is to promote health and prevent disease amongst children. This is achieved by means of the various activities which take place at the clinics.

At the infant welfare clinic

Infant welfare clinics are run by health sisters with the assistance of nursing sisters, staff nurses and, in some cases, community nurses. A health sister is a nurse who, after her training in general nursing and midwifery, undergoes a special training in public health nursing. She is therefore a nurse, a midwife and an expert in public health.

The main activities which take place at an infant welfare clinic are the registering of new cases, weighing and recording other measurements, interviewing mothers, examining babies, giving health education, immunising babies and treating minor ailments.

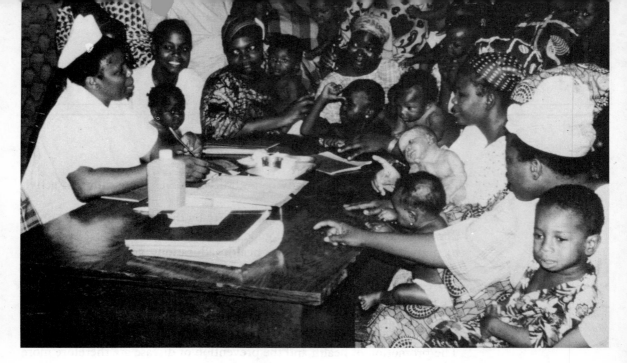

Fig 11.1   Registration at the infant welfare clinic.

Registration

Like all other clinics, an infant welfare clinic employs records clerks whose duties are to register and keep the records of all the children who attend the clinic.

The first thing you have to do when you take your baby to an infant welfare clinic for the first time is to register your baby at the registration desk, or counter, as the case may be. After your baby has been registered, the records clerk will give you your baby's **appointment card**. This card contains a fair amount of information designed to help and guide you. A typical appointment card is shown in Fig 11.2.

Fig 11.2   An infant welfare appointment card.

		Your next appointment is:				
		Date	Weight	Day	Date	Time
Surname _____ No_____						
First Name _____ Sex_____						
Date of Birth _____ Birth weight_____						
Address_____						
	Dates					
1 B.C.G.						
2 D.P.T	1_____					
	2_____					
	3_____					
3 Poliomyeitis	1_____					
	2_____					
	3_____					
4 Measles	1					
5 Small-pox	2_____					
6. Booster D.P.T.	1 / 2_____					
7. Booster Polio	1 / 2_____					

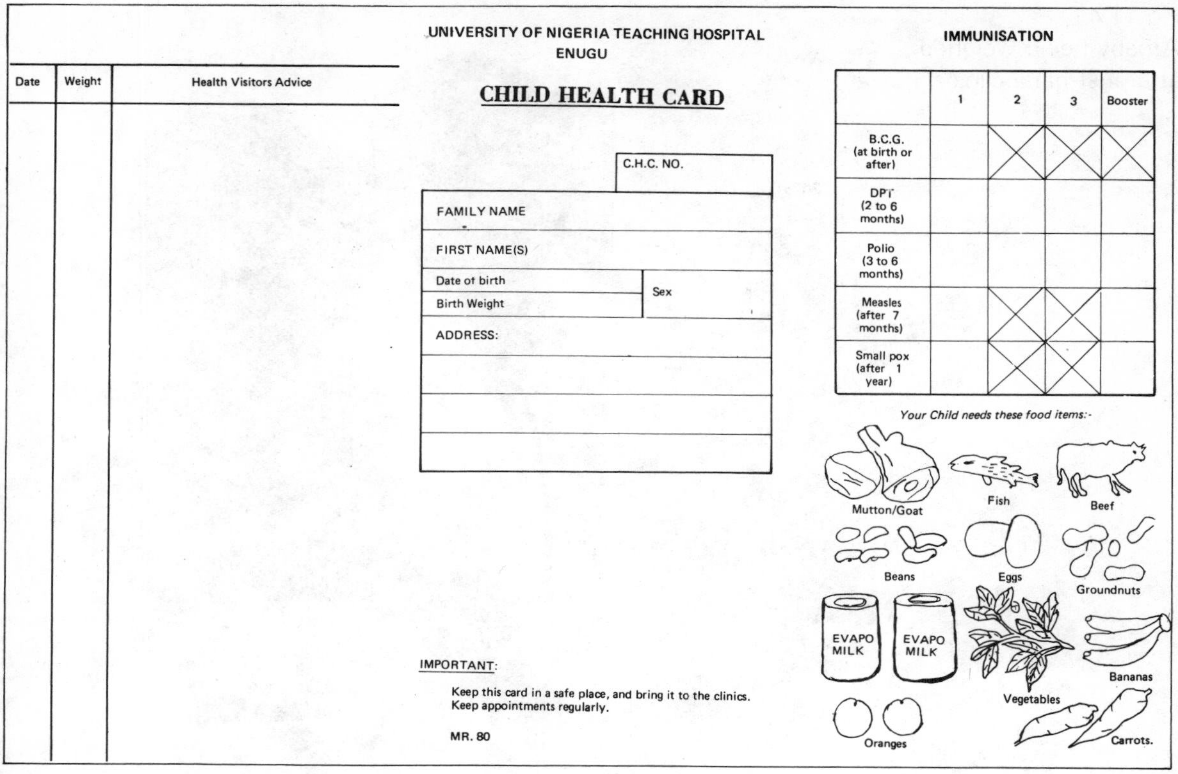

UNIVERSITY OF NIGERIA TEACHING HOSPITAL
ENUGU

CHILD HEALTH CARD

Date	Weight	Health Visitors Advice

C.H.C. NO.

FAMILY NAME

FIRST NAME(S)

Date of birth

Birth Weight

Sex

ADDRESS:

IMPORTANT:

Keep this card in a safe place, and bring it to the clinics.
Keep appointments regularly.

MR. 80

IMMUNISATION

	1	2	3	Booster
B.C.G. (at birth or after)				
DPT (2 to 6 months)				
Polio (3 to 6 months)				
Measles (after 7 months)				
Small pox (after 1 year)				

Your Child needs these food items:-

Mutton/Goat · Fish · Beef · Beans · Eggs · Groundnuts · EVAPO MILK · EVAPO MILK · Vegetables · Bananas · Oranges · Carrots.

Fig 11.3   An infant welfare record card.

The records clerk will also give you another much larger **record card**. This card will be used by the nursing staff to keep a record of your baby's progress. It is usually kept at the clinic but some clinics may allow you to keep it with your baby's appointment card. You are then expected to bring the two cards along with you whenever you attend the clinic. A typical record card is shown in Fig 11.3. As you can see, the section for recording your baby's weight is an important part of the record card.

When to register your baby

If your baby was delivered in a hospital or maternity home, the medical staff there will continue to follow your baby's progress until he is six weeks old. During that time, both of you will be expected to attend a special clinic at the hospital or maternity home. This clinic is known as a **post-natal clinic**. You will both be examined to ensure that all is well. After that, you will be told to go and register your baby at the infant welfare clinic nearest to you. You should do this as soon as possible.

If you did not register for antenatal care at a hospital or maternity home (as you should have done), and your baby was delivered at home, you should register your baby at the nearest infant welfare clinic before he is one week old. This is because your baby should receive his first immunisation during the first week of his life. It is also important that medically qualified personnel should keep an eye on your baby from birth.

97

Fig 11.4
A baby being weighed
at a post-natal clinic.

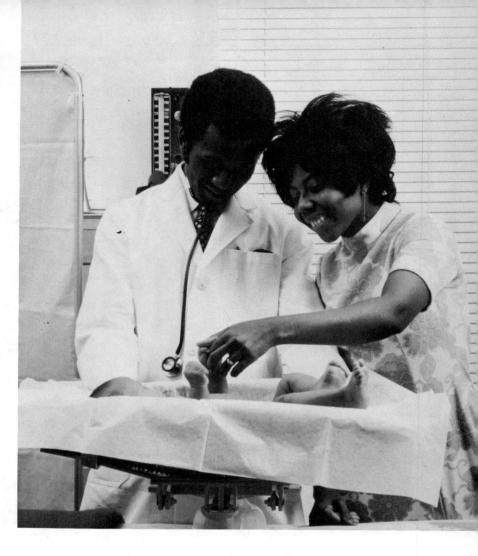

Some infant welfare clinics only accept babies from the age of three months, when the major part of their immunisation treatment is expected to start. However, many mothers require medical help and guidance when their babies are less than three months old. This applies particularly to mothers who did not have proper antenatal care and who delivered their babies at home. Mothers should be encouraged to register their babies as soon as possible after delivery.

Weighing and other measurements

Every infant welfare clinic has special scales for measuring a baby's weight. Some clinics also take a note of the baby's height and, occasionally, other measurements as well. The purpose of all these measurements is to ensure that your baby is growing normally. The results are entered in a special column on the record card (and sometimes on the appointment card as well) or on the weight chart on the record card. It is clearer to show a child's progress in the form of a chart rather than as a series of figures in

98

a column. This is because a chart shows the child's progress at a glance. Some weight charts show weight (and sometimes height) curves for the average normal baby so that you can compare your baby's actual measurements with those to be expected. It is important for every mother to keep a careful note of her baby's progress in gaining weight so that she will notice any failure to gain weight at an early stage (see page 109).

Interviewing the mother

The health sister and her assistants at the infant welfare clinic hold a private interview with each mother which should take the form of an informal and friendly chat. Its purpose is to give the mother an opportunity to discuss with the sister or nurse any medical problems she may have and to receive help and guidance.

Do not hesitate to ask the nursing staff about anything concerning the health of your baby, no matter how trivial you may think it is. This is particularly important if the baby is your first and you are not yet experienced in child care. You should ask for the opinion of the staff before acting on any other medical advice which you may have received from friends and relations. Bad advice from well-meaning friends and relations has been the cause of tragedies which could have been avoided.

General examination

After your interview, the sister or staff nurse will examine the baby. The purpose of this examination is to look for any signs of disease or disability so that something can be done about them as early as possible.

While examining the baby, the staff nurse may ask you some questions. You should answer her questions as truthfully as you can without keeping any information back.

Health education

This is a very important facility offered by the infant welfare clinic. The role of health education in promoting health and preventing disease cannot be over-emphasised, especially where people still have superstitions about various health matters. Every mother who attends an infant welfare clinic should listen very carefully to the health education lectures and learn as much as she can.

Health education consists of simple lectures on health. The waiting section in the clinic may also be used as a lecture hall as can be seen in Fig 11.1. The talks are most useful when accompanied by practical demonstrations. The clinic should also be provided with cooking facilities for food demonstrations.

Immunisation

Immunisation, which is also popularly called **vaccination**, involves the administration of a vaccine to an individual to protect the individual against a particular disease or infection (see page 124).

Vaccines are made from micro-organisms which are either bacteria or viruses. Some vaccines contain living micro-organisms but in a very weak

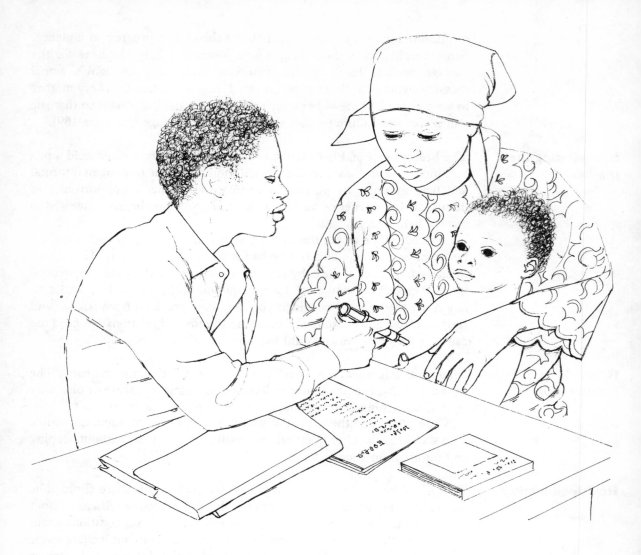

Fig 11.5   Immunisation at the clinic.

and harmless form. They are called live vaccines. Others, referred to as dead or killed vaccines, contain extracts from dead micro-organisms.

When a vaccine is introduced into the body, it causes the body to produce antibodies. These antibodies protect the individual against the disease caused by the micro-organism from which the vaccine has been made.

Antibodies are highly complex protein substances whose job in the body is to prevent or fight disease. Newborn babies receive antibodies from their mothers while in the womb and continue to receive them through breast milk.

| **Vaccines used in infant welfare clinics** | Modern science has not been able to produce vaccines to fight against *all* harmful micro-organisms. However, it has been able to make vaccines which fight against some very important diseases. The vaccines which are available in infant welfare clinics are the BCG, DTP, polio, measles and smallpox vaccines. |

BCG vaccine

This vaccine protects against tuberculosis and is given by means of an injection into the skin of the right shoulder. A single injection is usually sufficient to protect the individual. A small swelling or nodule appears about three weeks after the injection has been given. This nodule may later become a small ulcer which will slowly heal. Sometimes the glands in the armpit also become enlarged but this should not cause any alarm.

DTP vaccine

This vaccine is also known as the triple vaccine as it is a mixture of three different vaccines. These are the diphtheria, tetanus, and whooping cough (pertussis) vaccines.

DTP immunisation protects against diphtheria, tetanus and whooping cough and is given by means of an injection into the muscles of the buttocks. More than one injection is necessary to produce an adequate amount of antibodies.

Polio vaccine

There are two types of polio vaccine. One type contains live polio organisms and is given by mouth in the form of drops. The other type contains dead polio organisms and is given by an injection into the muscles of the buttocks. The vaccine given by mouth is the one generally preferred in most infant welfare clinics, probably because it is cheaper than the other type of vaccine and is easier to administer as it does not have to be given by means of an injection.

Measles vaccine

This vaccine contains living measles organisms. It is given by means of injection under the skin of the buttocks. It is one of the most useful vaccines which has so far been produced. Mothers whose infants have suffered from measles will appreciate the value of this vaccine.

Occasionally, the vaccine causes a mild form of measles but this should not cause alarm. This happens when the power of the measles organisms in the vaccine has not been completely destroyed.

Smallpox vaccine

This vaccine is also known as **vaccinia**. It is a live vaccine and is given in a rather peculiar manner. Several pinpricks are made with a sharp needle through a drop of the vaccine on the skin of the left shoulder. When the vaccine is given for the first time, the process is known as the **primary vaccination**. Primary vaccinations always cause a lot of soreness and reaction and leave a permanent scar. A sore from a smallpox vaccination may cause irritation but must be left strictly alone and must not be touched or scratched. Smallpox vaccination has been suspended in the last few years, because the disease has been virtually eliminated from the world. This has been achieved entirely through immunisation.

Schedule for immunisations

Infants are immunised according to a special schedule. This schedule has been carefully worked out to produce the best results. It is important for all mothers to realise this because some people wrongly believe that

101

Baby's age	Vaccines given	Notes
First week of life	BCG	Should be given before the mother is discharged from the hospital or maternity home after confinement.
3 months	DTP — 1st dose Polio — 1st dose	
4 months	DTP — 2nd dose Polio — 2nd dose	
5 months	DTP — 3rd dose Polio — 3rd dose	
7 to 9 months	Measles	Some clinics give two doses, one at 6 months and another at 12 months.
18 months	DTP — 4th dose (first booster) Polio — 4th dose (first booster)	
5 years	DTP — 5th dose (second booster) Polio — 5th dose (second booster)	

Fig 11.6   Immunisation schedule.

vaccines can be given in any order and at any time. Fig 11.6 shows the schedule which must be followed.

Complications

There are very few complications or side effects caused by immunisation and most of these are avoidable. The following are the main complications which can occur.

Fever

This is by far the most common side effect of immunisation. It may arise a few days after immunisation but it will not be a high fever and will usually subside with the aid of a little aspirin or a similar drug. Mothers should be warned that a fever may occur and be supplied with some junior aspirin tablets or syrup whenever their babies are immunised (see page 119).

Occasionally, the fever is severe and troublesome but this is very unusual. The whooping cough vaccine contained in the DTP vaccine is usually the cause of the fever.

Infection

The injection area may become infected causing pain, redness and a swelling of the area. The infection results from inadequate cleaning of the area before and after the injection and can easily be avoided if the nurse who gives the injection and the mother who looks after the child both observe absolute cleanliness.

Sometimes an infection forms an abscess. This happens most often when the treatment of the infection is not started early enough. At the least sign of infection, the child should be taken to the clinic immediately for treatment.

Sterile abscess A sterile abscess is the swelling which may develop following an injection of vaccine. It occurs mainly with DTP immunisation. The swelling results from the failure of the vaccine to be absorbed into the bloodstream. The vaccine remains at the injection site and attracts more fluid to itself.

The swelling is not infected and is therefore not a true abscess and will eventually disappear without any treatment.

Gland enlargement This occurs mainly with BCG immunisation. The glands in the armpit may become quite large and look rather frightening but they will also eventually disappear without the necessity for any treatment.

Measles rash About ten days after the measles immunisation, a mild form of measles rash may appear on the infant's body and may be accompanied by a fever. This type of reaction is caused by the live virus in the measles vaccine. It does not usually cause the infant any harm and all traces of illness will subside within a few days. The fever and any discomfort from the rash can be relieved with junior aspirin and calamine lotion.

Convulsions These are by far the most serious of the side effects of immunisation. Fortunately, they are also the least common and again it is the whooping cough vaccine which is mainly responsible.

When not to immunise Immunisation is witheld only under certain circumstances, the most common of which are outlined here.

1. If the baby already has a fever or some other sign of illness such as a cough or diarrhoea he should not be immunised until he is well again. The reason for this is that the child may react unfavourably to immunisation and it may then be very difficult to know how much of his illness is due to his original disease and how much is due to the immunisation.

   Immunisation should continue as soon as the child is well again.

2. If a child reacted to the first DTP vaccination by having a severe fever, he should not be given any more of the vaccine. In some countries, such a child would be given a DT vaccine which contains only the diphtheria and tetanus vaccines but this vaccine is not yet available in African countries.

3. A child who has had convulsions in the past should not be given a DTP immunisation but he could be given the DT vaccine if it is available.

4. A child who has had measles does not need a measles immunisation because the illness itself will usually give him adequate protection against a second attack.

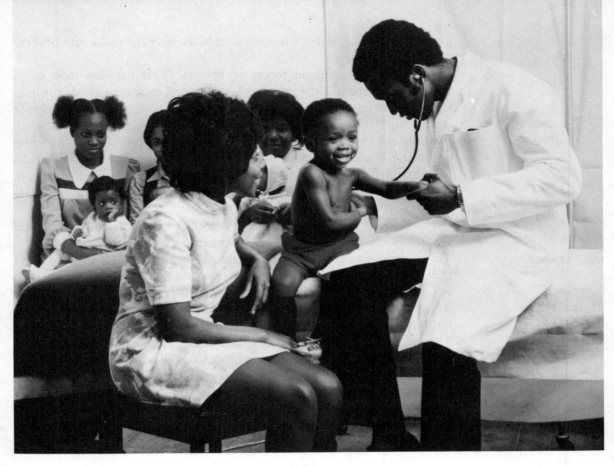

Fig 11.7   Many clinics have a visiting doctor.

Treatment

Most infant welfare clinics treat minor childhood ailments. This is a good thing because early treatment prevents the illness from getting worse. Also, the mother is saved the trouble of taking her child to another clinic for special treatment.

Besides treating minor ailments, the clinic staff will also refer medical problems to the appropriate medical department for treatment. Ideally, an infant welfare clinic should have a doctor who visits at least once a week and to whom the medical problems would be referred in the first instance. Unfortunately, this is not usually possible in areas where doctors are few and far between.

The importance of infant welfare clinics

The services provided by all infant welfare clinics are entirely free. This is a deliberate policy on the part of the authorities, who are aware of the importance of these clinics, and is designed to encourage mothers to take their babies to the clinics. Mothers have only themselves to blame if they do not make the best possible use of the infant welfare clinic nearest to them.

Modern medicine has not been able to provide a cure for some very harmful diseases. It has therefore tried to investigate whether such diseases can be eliminated by immunisation. Diseases such as measles, whooping cough and polio are notable examples. Quite apart from the useful advice and guidance which a mother can receive at an infant welfare clinic, it is in the mother's interest that her baby should be protected from diseases, especially from those for which there is no cure as yet.

12

Signs of illness and failure to thrive

Newborn babies and very young children react to many illnesses in a similar manner, which makes it difficult to diagnose what is wrong. In addition, illnesses in very young children and babies tend to progress rapidly unless treatment is started promptly. It is therefore very important for mothers to be able to recognise early signs of illness in newborn babies and young children so that they can do something about the illness in good time.

Early signs of illness

The following are the more common early signs of illness in newborn babies and young children.

Refusal to feed

Healthy infants have a good appetite. Refusal to feed is probably the commonest and most important early sign of illness in newborn babies and young children. When asking a mother about her baby's illness, one of the first things a doctor wants to know is how well the baby has been feeding.

On the other hand, if you think that your baby is ill even though he is eating well, he is probably not as ill as you imagine.

Dullness

The medical term for dullness is *apathy*. Healthy infants, including newborns, should be alert when they are awake. If their behaviour changes so that they become more subdued than normal, something is probably wrong.

Irritability

An infant may become fretful and irritable for many reasons. He may be tired, hungry, uncomfortable or may be feeling unwell. If he is not feeling well he will dislike any form of handling and want to be left alone. Any attempt to carry him will only make him cry. Irritability is a prominent early sign of certain diseases including brain infections.

Excessive crying

Crying is the main method by which infants express their needs. Normally, an infant will stop crying when his needs have been satisfied but sometimes he may continue to cry for no obvious reason.

Excessive crying may be due to bad temper but it may also be a sign that something is wrong. Infants who are ill cry because they do not feel well or because they are in pain. Illnesses which often cause excessive crying in infants include ear infections, which can cause severe earache, throat infections, which can cause sore throats, meningitis, a brain infection which causes severe headaches, osteomyelitis (a bone infection), and some urinary diseases which cause discomfort when the child urinates.

Excessive sleepiness

Although a mother will tend to regard a newborn baby who gives little trouble and sleeps most of the time as a 'good' baby, such a baby may not actually be 'good' as far as his health is concerned.

Excessive sleepiness often goes hand in hand with apathy. Infants who sleep because they are ill are also dull when they are awake. On the other hand, if a baby sleeps for much of the time but is alert and active when he is awake, then he is probably quite healthy.

Vomiting

This is a very common sign of illness and is often the first sign that something is wrong.

Vomiting may occur during, after or between feeds. If it coincides with feeding, then all the feed will be vomited out. If persistent, this will lead to a rapid loss of weight unless the illness can be brought under control quickly.

Vomiting should not be confused with regurgitation, when the infant brings up some of his recent feed which then spills out of his mouth. This often happens, particularly during weaning, and is perfectly normal.

There are several causes of vomiting, one of which is **gastro-enteritis** (see page 122). If the child starts projectile vomiting, then he should be taken to a doctor immediately.

Fever

The part of the brain which regulates the temperature of the body is known as the temperature regulating centre. In newborn babies and very young children the temperature regulating centre is not fully developed and they will tend to adopt the temperature of their surroundings.

Illness can easily affect the temperature regulating centre, causing a rapid rise in the infant's temperature and we say that the child has a fever (see page 119). What is more, the child's temperature may become quite high in a very short time causing a high fever, and may lead to convulsions (see page 128). Fortunately, young children withstand high temperatures better than older children and adults do but their skin temperature may not reflect their true body temperature. The correct temperature of a sick baby can *only* be determined by using a special **thermometer** *which must be used correctly* (see page 120).

Coldness of the body

When the temperature regulating centre is damaged by illness, it may become unable to maintain the body temperature which will then rapidly fall. This happens mainly with severe infections and can be dangerous. However, if the child has **hypothermia**, as the condition is medically known, the whole body will become cold and not just the arms and legs.

Changes in skin colour

Most African babies are pinkish in colour at birth. The ears are the only parts of the body which are likely to give a true picture of a newborn's final skin colour.

Sudden changes in skin colour are important and are early signs of illness in newborn babies. The baby's skin may become paler, darker, or yellowish in colour. The yellowish colour is a sign of jaundice.

Twitching

This means the sudden and irregular movements of individual muscles in different parts of the baby's body. These should not be confused with the jerking movements which are a baby's normal reaction to a sudden loud noise or bang. Twitching is a serious sign which indicates that an illness has affected the brain. It is usually preceded by a high fever and can lead to convulsions, which are a more serious condition.

Convulsions

These are frightening, jerky movements of the whole body which are often accompanied by a rolling of the eyes. They may also be accompanied by a throaty and noisy type of breathing.

Convulsions may be caused by disorderly activity of the brain. Many illnesses affect the brain and cause it to behave in this disorderly manner (see also page 128).

What to do

Although mothers can easily recognise and treat some disorders such as diarrhoea (see page 116) or fever (see page 119) simply by knowing what to do to help their sick baby, some of the most difficult problems which doctors and nurses have to deal with are *advanced* cases of illness which have been brought in too late for treatment. Many sick children die simply because they were not brought in for treatment early enough. Some people foolishly prefer to buy drugs themselves from a chemist's shop, market stall or drug pedlar and treat their children themselves. This is a very dangerous practice for several reasons. First of all, such people are not trained to recognise and diagnose illnesses correctly with the result that they do not actually know what they are treating, although they may think that they do. Secondly, they do not know the correct dosages of the drugs they are giving or what precautions to take. Thirdly, many dangerous micro-organisms are becoming resistant to drugs because these drugs are used so extensively and often needlessly. In many countries, drugs are sold only on a doctor's prescription so that doctors can keep a check on the drugs used by their patients.

If you suspect that your baby is ill and you are not sure how to treat him, you should take him to the nearest hospital, health centre, clinic or maternity home. Illness in very young children tends to get worse rapidly if not promptly treated. You should therefore not delay as it is dangerous to do so. *Doctors or nurses will be less angry with you for bringing a healthy baby to see them than they will be if you allow the baby's illness to become serious before you take him to them for treatment.*

Failure to thrive

This simply means a failure to gain weight. Sometimes it is a sign that a child's illness is slowing him down and so the cause must be found quickly, possibly with the help of some medical tests. An important function of infant welfare clinics is to spot the child who is not gaining weight satisfactorily so that something can be done about it in time to prevent serious damage to the child's health. A mother must study her baby's weight chart (see page 99) very carefully to watch for early signs of illness.

Failure to thrive has several causes. The four most common of these are mentioned here.

Inadequate feeding

This is the most common cause of failure to thrive because if the infant is not fed adequately he simply does not receive enough nourishment. There are several reasons why an infant might not be fed adequately. First of all, there may not be enough breast milk for the baby. Secondly, when the infant has been weaned off the breast and is on a full adult diet, the parents may not realise that milk feeds should be continued (see Chapter 8) and may be too poor to afford to buy enough food. Lastly, the parents may not be aware of the importance of providing a balanced diet (see Chapter 7), even though they can afford to buy enough food. Young couples, who are just beginning to have children, are sometimes unaware of the importance of correct infant-feeding.

If not taken care of in time, poor feeding can eventually lead to malnutrition, or **kwashiorkor**, a disease which eventually develops if a child does not have enough protein in his diet.

Infections

An infection can lead to a failure to thrive in many ways. Firstly, it tends to suppress the child's appetite so that the child does not eat enough. Secondly, the child may vomit or have diarrhoea, leading to the loss of whatever food he has managed to eat. Thirdly, the micro-organism causing the infection may also take food substances from the patient's body. All of these conditions cause the child to lose weight.

Infections are most common among children who grow up in unhygienic conditions. To make matters worse, repeated infections usually go hand in hand with poor feeding because a lack of proper nourishment will lower the body's resistance to infection.

Infections which often lead to failure to thrive include malaria, gastro-enteritis (diarrhoea and vomiting) (see page 122), measles and tuberculosis.

Neglect or maternal deprivation

Neglect of a growing infant by his mother is unfortunately becoming more common. Because of changes caused by modern society, many mothers now work outside the family home leaving their children in the care of child-minders. When a working mother returns home in the evening, she may be too tired to take proper care of her child and so the child is deprived of his mother's love and attention.

Infants are very sensitive and feel a great sense of loss if they are deprived of their mother's love. They can become depressed and unhappy and, even if they do manage to eat enough, they simply do not gain weight which shows how much the mind can influence the body!

An infant who is deprived of his mother's love is said to be suffering from maternal deprivation. **Paediatricians** and other child health workers are becoming concerned about the increasing number of cases of maternal deprivation which they meet.

Poor organ development (congenital abnormality)

Something may go wrong with the development of a baby while he is still in the womb. This often occurs during the first three months of pregnancy. The organs of the body which are most often affected in this way are the heart, limbs, brain and kidneys. The affected organ may then be unable to function properly and may show this by causing a failure to thrive.

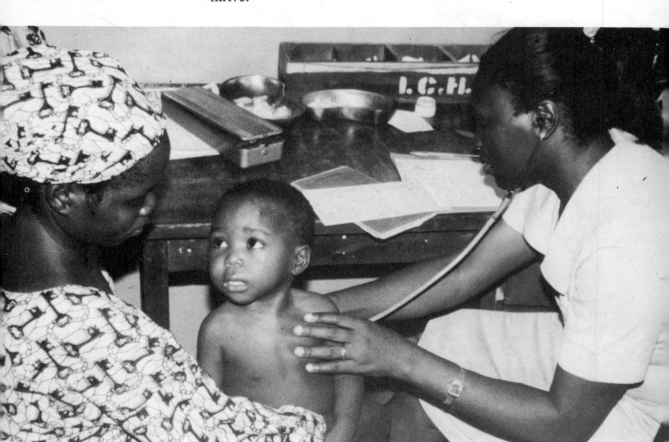

Fig 12.1   A sick child being examined at a clinic.

What to do

It is clear that a proper examination will be necessary to find out the cause of a failure to thrive but this does not necessarily mean that the child must undergo complicated medical tests. Each case will have to be dealt with on an individual basis.

If you feel that your baby is not growing as he should, you should take him to the infant welfare clinic which you should have been attending for his immunisations and general care. You could, alternatively, take him to the nearest hospital.

Most cases of failure to thrive are caused by poor feeding or by infections, some of which have already been mentioned. Your infant welfare clinic should be able to take care of the problem for you but if the staff at the clinic think that it is necessary to do so, they will refer your child to a doctor for further examination and treatment.

13

Common illnessess and conditions in newborn babies

Because their organs are not fully developed, newborn babies are very susceptible to illness. Unfortunately, maturity is a process which takes time and nothing can be done to hasten it. Newborn infants should not be handled by anyone with any illness, no matter how mild.

Common illnesses

There are certain illnesses to which newborn babies are particularly susceptible and which are found only in infants. The most common of these are outlined here.

Failure to breathe at birth

This is known as **asphyxia of the newborn**. It usually occurs in infants born after a prolonged or difficult labour. The infant does not cry immediately after birth and his skin may be dark blue, in which case he has blue asphyxia, or pale in colour, in which case he has white asphyxia. In the case of blue asphyxia, the infant lacks only oxygen whereas in white asphyxia, lack of oxygen is accompanied by the failure of the heart to pump out blood and this is therefore a much more serious condition.

The brain is more sensitive to lack of oxygen than any other organ in the body. Failure to treat asphyxia of the newborn promptly may cause permanent brain damage, if the infant survives at all. For this reason, mothers who have had a prolonged or difficult labour in the past should always have their babies in hospital.

Birth injury

As with asphyxia of the newborn, birth injury occurs mainly in infants who are born after a difficult delivery. The infants may suffer from different kinds of injury during delivery of which the following are the more common.

Bleeding

Bleeding mainly affects the scalp and the eyes. Bleeding under the scalp causes a swelling on one or both sides of the head. The edges of the swelling are hard while the centre is soft and this may cause the swelling to be mistaken for a fracture. It disappears slowly over a period of two to four weeks, does not require any treatment and should be left completely alone.

Bleeding in the eyes may be mild, affecting only a small part of one or both eyes, or it may be extensive and alarming. Whatever the extent of the bleeding, it should be left strictly alone. This, also, will clear slowly of its own accord.

Nerve injuries	These mainly affect the arms. Nerves may be damaged if considerable pressure is applied to one side of the infant's neck during delivery. The arm on that side of the body may then become paralysed causing it to hang limply at the infant's side. He should be taken to a doctor for treatment without delay.
Bone fractures	These may occur if too much force is used during delivery. The collar bone is the bone most often affected. A fracture of the collar bone causes the arm on the same side of the body as the fractured bone to hang limply looking as if it is paralysed. The fracture may only be noticed when a lump appears at the site of the fracture. This consists of new bone which forms when the fracture begins to heal.

The bones of an arm or leg may also fracture. *All fractures should be taken to a doctor for prompt treatment.*

Vomiting

During delivery, the infant may swallow some of the amniotic fluid which surrounded him in the womb. This irritates the child's stomach and causes vomiting but this is not usually serious and is treated, if necessary, by washing out the stomach with sterile water. If the vomiting is serious, and persists after the stomach has been washed out, then there is probably a more serious underlying cause such as an obstruction of the intestines or an infection. In such a case, you must take your baby to a hospital or clinic without delay.

Sticky eyes

Amniotic fluid can also irritate the infant's eyes. If it enters the baby's eyes during delivery, it can cause a mild inflammation of the eyes. This produces a slight, colourless discharge which causes the eyelids to stick together during sleep. The discharge is most noticeable when the infant wakes up in the morning. The eyes clear up quickly if treated with mild antiseptic eye lotion.

Wind colic

Not all paediatricians believe that too much wind can cause abdominal colic in infants. Those who do, believe that failing to make an infant bring up the excess wind after breast-feeding leads to wind colic, which makes the infant cry. The majority of mothers also believe that excessive crying in infants is often caused by abdominal pain. However, most of them wrongly blame the umbilicus for causing the pain and so do not realise that the pain may be cause by wind colic.

Many 'anti-colic' or gripe medicines are available in shops and markets. Some of them are modern drugs while others are traditional medicines. It is important for mothers to know that some of the highly advertised traditional gripe medicines have been the cause of serious illness in infants. A mother should *not* give her baby these medicines without seeking a doctor's advice. An infant who cries excessively should be taken to a doctor for a check-up and his mother should *not* assume that his excessive crying means that he has wind colic. To do so may cause further harm to the baby.

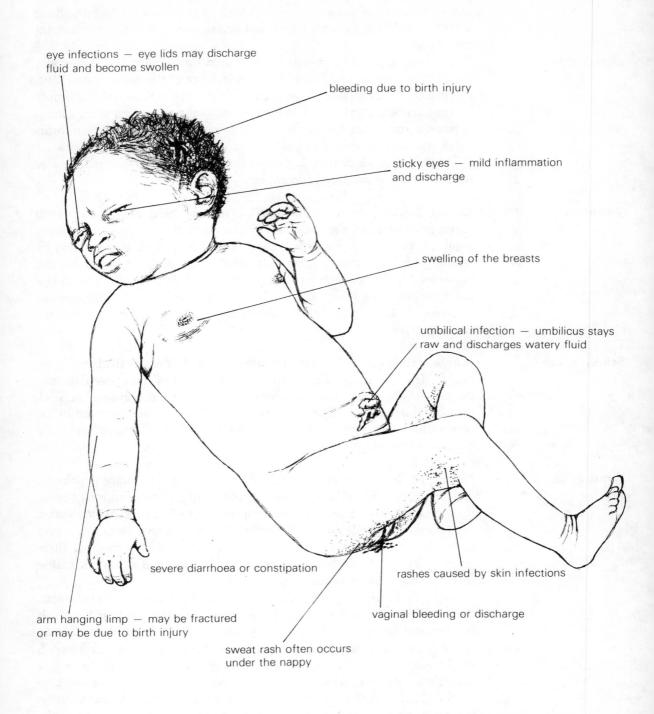

eye infections — eye lids may discharge
fluid and become swollen

bleeding due to birth injury

sticky eyes — mild inflammation
and discharge

swelling of the breasts

umbilical infection — umbilicus stays
raw and discharges watery fluid

severe diarrhoea or constipation

rashes caused by skin infections

arm hanging limp — may be fractured
or may be due to birth injury

vaginal bleeding or discharge

sweat rash often occurs
under the nappy

Fig 13.1   Symptoms of some illnesses in newborn babies.

Umbilical infection   Failure to keep the umbilical area clean, particularly after the cord has fallen off, often causes an infection. Because of its close link with the blood and the liver, an infected umbilicus may quickly cause blood or liver infections which would have serious consequences. If the umbilical infection is caused by the tetanus germ the infant may develop tetanus, a dangerous disease in newborn infants. Neonatal tetanus, as the disease is known, will be discussed later in this chapter.

An infected umbilicus remains raw and does not heal. It may discharge pus or a watery fluid which is sometimes blood-stained. The infected area should be cleaned two or three times a day with soap and water, dried with a little methylated spirit, and then painted with an antiseptic solution such as gentian violet until the cord heals and falls off. The umbilicus should be protected with a dressing held in place by a bandage (see page 18) until the cord falls off. There is no need for a dressing or bandage after the cord has fallen off. These measures are usually adequate for mild cases but more serious cases will require antibiotics which are best prescribed by a doctor.

Skin infections   Infections of the skin can take various forms which are known by different names including boils, abscesses, septic rashes and ulcers. They are all caused by germs passed on to the infant from those who handle him. A mother with any ulcers or septic spots on her hands can cause skin infections by rubbing the germs into the child's skin. For this reason, anyone who handles a baby must ensure that strict hygiene has been observed so that their hands are absolutely clean and free from infection. If mild skin infections in newborn babies are not promptly treated they may lead to serious complications such as blood-poisoning (**septicaemia**).

One of the most common skin infections is known as **impetigo**. This infection begins as a red spot which becomes a small blister within a few hours. The fluid in the blister is clear at first so that the affected area resembles a burn. However, the fluid quickly turns to pus and the blister then ruptures to leave a shallow ulcer. Impetigo is often mistaken for sweat rash. Sweat rash and milia rash will be discussed later in this chapter.

The treatment of skin infections includes the use of antibiotic sprays and creams, frequent bathing with antiseptic soap and, in some cases, the application of an antiseptic lotion to the skin. *The best person to advise on treatment is a doctor or qualified nurse.*

Eye infections   If the eyes are infected they become inflamed and red in colour. They produce a discharge which is watery at first but soon turns to pus. In severe cases, the eyelids become so swollen that it is difficult to see the eyes at all.

Eye infections are usually caused by a contamination of the eyes during birth. This contamination may come from the mother's birth canal or from the fingers of those who helped at the birth. The eyes are treated by washing three to four times a day with antiseptic or antibiotic eye drops.

Severe cases will require vigorous treatment with an antibiotic prescribed by a doctor. If only one eye is infected, the infant should lie with the affected eye *nearest* the pillow. This will prevent the discharge from flowing into the healthy eye.

Blood infection

This is blood-poisoning and is known as septicaemia. It is a very dangerous condition which is best treated in hospital. It often results from skin or umbilical infections. Unfortunately, there are no special signs by which septicaemia can be recognised in newborn babies. This is why it is so important to take a baby to a doctor as soon as any signs of illness are noticed. When treating septicaemia, the germ responsible is identified through special blood tests. This is to find out which antibiotic drugs should be used. The drugs are given by an injection into the muscles of the buttocks or directly into the bloodstream.

Catarrh

Although catarrh is usually a mild infection, causing little concern in older children and adults, it is a potentially dangerous infection in a newborn infant. The tiny nostrils of the infant can easily become blocked, making it difficult for him to breathe or feed properly. In this case, the baby's nose should be gently wiped to remove as much catarrh as possible before feeding.

Persistent catarrh in newborn babies has a tendency to develop quickly into pneumonia and so must be promptly treated by a doctor.

Pneumonia

This is another dangerous disease in newborn infants and often results from catarrh which was not treated promptly. The well-known signs of pneumonia such as coughing and fast breathing may not occur in an infant with the result that the mother and others are misled.

Most mothers know that exposing an infant to cold and damp weather makes him liable to catch catarrh and then pneumonia. However, it is not generally known that the actual infection can be spread to the infant by someone who has handled the infant and has catarrh or a cough. *Anyone with a cold or a cough should stay away from young infants.*

Diarrhoea

Diarrhoea used to be uncommon in newborn infants because they were fed only on breast milk. In recent times, artificial feeding has become more widespread and unfortunately the precautions detailed in Chapter 4 are not always carried out. This has led to an increase in diarrhoea amongst children whose artificial feeds *have not been properly prepared*. Diarrhoea is dangerous in all children but is particularly dangerous in newborn infants. It is usually accompanied by a rapid loss of weight and, in severe cases, the infant may look dry and shrivelled due to a loss of water from the body. A mother can try to remedy this by frequently giving her baby water with sugar and a little salt in it. If the diarrhoea continues for more than a day she should take her baby to a doctor. As was mentioned in Chapter 3, colostrum (the first milk produced by the mother's breasts after confinement) causes frequent bowel motions in some infants but *this is not true diarrhoea* and the infant will continue to gain weight.

Constipation

A newborn infant will usually have frequent bowel motions. Some newborn babies, however, do not open their bowels frequently; but when they do the stool is quite soft and normal. If the baby has constipation, the stool is hard and is often difficult to pass.

Constipation is not common in infants fed entirely on the breast but occurs more often in infants fed with artificial milk. An infant who is prone to constipation should be given extra water between feeds. As soon as he is one month old, orange juice and other fruit juices can be added to his diet. These will help to soften his stool and prevent constipation.

Tetanus

Tetanus in newborn infants is known as neonatal tetanus. The signs of tetanus are the same in newborn babies as in older children and adults. The affected newborn will be unable to open his mouth, his whole body will have repeated contractions and his neck, trunk and limbs will become rigid. Any form of disturbance, including noise or bright light, will bring on the contractions.

Doctors are only able to save the lives of about fifty per cent of older children and adults suffering from tetanus and in the case of newborn infants only about five to ten per cent of those with tetanus are saved. It is therefore extremely important to prevent tetanus in newborn infants. Tetanus is prevented by immunising the mother during pregnancy and by keeping the newborn's umbilicus and circumcision wounds scrupulously clean. Newborns whose mothers were not immunised against tetanus during pregnancy should be given an **anti-tetanus serum** at birth.

Other common conditions

There are some other conditions which occur quite often in newborn infants and are usually quite harmless. Some of the more common ones are mentioned here.

Extra digits

These usually bear little or no resemblance to normal fingers or toes. An extra digit is attached to the side of the little finger or toe of one or both hands or feet. It is often nothing more than a small lump of flesh. The midwife deals with it by tying a piece of cotton thread tightly round the base of the lump to cut off the blood supply to it. Within a few days, it will shrivel and fall off. However if the extra digit is more than merely a small lump of flesh, it should not be tied off but should be shown to a doctor.

Birthmarks

These can be of different colours, shapes and forms and are known by various names. Some birthmarks have hair on them.

Most birthmarks do not change in any way as the infant grows older. If a birthmark increases in size, or begins to change in some other way, then it should be examined by a doctor. A birthmark which increases in size is usually caused by a collection of abnormal blood vessels and may have to be treated. Treatment may also be needed for cosmetic reasons if a birthmark is unsightly.

Peeling skin

Mild peeling of the skin occurs during the second or third week of life in many newborn infants. Occasionally, the peeling of the skin is extensive and a little alarming. This occurs mainly in infants who were born well after their expected date of birth. Post-mature infants, as these infants are known, have dry wrinkled skin which may peel off in large segments. The new skin which is underneath the peeling skin is quite normal and healthy.

Milia rash and sweat rash

Milia rash is a finely spotted rash which bears little resemblance to impetigo but is often confused with it. In milia rash, the individual spots are tiny and each spot has a creamy centre which is quite hard and can be squeezed out using the fingers. There are no signs of inflammation as shown by redness or tenderness of the skin. The rash disappears slowly without any treatment.

Sweat rash is also finely spotted. Each spot contains a clear liquid which is actually sweat. The rash develops as a result of the way in which the newborn infant perspires. Instead of sweat lying on the surface of the skin, it becomes embedded in the skin. Like milia rash, sweat rash can also be confused with impetigo.

Swelling of the breasts

The breasts sometimes become enlarged in newborn babies and may even secrete milk. The enlargement is caused by chemical substances which the infant received from his mother while he was in the womb. The substances are known as oestrogens and were produced by the mother's ovaries. The infant slowly eliminates the oestrogens from his body, so reducing the enlargement gradually until it disappears completely.

The enlarged breasts do not need any treatment and should be left alone. Any form of interference is liable to result in an infection which frequently leads to the formation of an abscess.

Vaginal discharge or bleeding

The same oestrogens which cause breast enlargement in newborns of both sexes are responsible for a vaginal discharge which is sometimes seen in newborn baby girls. The oestrogens act on the infant's genital organs exactly as they do in adult females and cause a white, inoffensive vaginal discharge. Instead of having a vaginal discharge, the infant may react with 'menstrual' bleeding.

Both the vaginal discharge and bleeding clear up within a few days and do not require any treatment but if they persist you should contact a doctor.

14 Common illnesses in young children

The illnesses from which people suffer are greatly influenced by the environment in which they live. The illnesses which are most common in a community therefore vary from one part of the world to another.

Environmental factors which are important in determining the pattern of disease in any community include climate, the presence of parasites, pests and micro-organisms, nutrition and cultural beliefs and practices. How some of these factors influence the health of the community has already been discussed earlier in the book.

Many children grow up in an unhygienic environment and eat a predominantly starchy diet. The illnesses from which these children suffer will reflect their environment.

Fever

Many illnesses can cause a child to have a fever. It is not an illness itself but is a symptom of many different illnesses. A fever occurs when the body temperature is higher than normal (which is 37°C). If the child's temperature is above 39°C then he has a high fever, which may be dangerous. Body temperature is measured using a thermometer (see page 120).

If a child has a fever the following precautions should be taken.
1. Undress the child and leave him uncovered.
2. Sponge him gently with cool water to lower his temperature.
3. Try to encourage him to drink plenty of water, fruit juice or other liquid. For young babies, remember to use boiled water.
4. A little junior aspirin or paracetamol may help to reduce the fever but *only use these if you are sure of the correct dosage.* No drug at all is much better than too much.
5. Take the child to the doctor as soon as possible.

The 'top ten' diseases

The ten most frequent types of illness amongst the children in any community are responsible for more than ninety per cent of the illnesses from which they suffer. Consequently, if we concentrate on preventing these 'top ten' diseases the health of the children will improve greatly.

The ten most common types of illness amongst children in most parts of the tropics are described in this chapter.

Using a thermometer

A thermometer is used to measure body temperature. You should be able to buy one in a local chemist's shop.

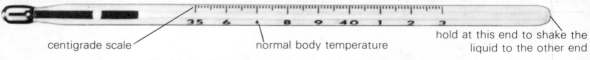

centigrade scale

normal body temperature

hold at this end to shake the liquid to the other end

Fig 14.1   Thermometer with a Centigrade (C) scale.

To use a thermometer correctly you must do the following.
1. Clean it well with soap and water.
2. Shake it hard holding it at the end shown above.
3. Place the thermometer under the baby's arm, in the armpit, holding the baby's arm down to keep the thermometer in position.
   Doctors and nurses usually place the thermometer in the baby's anus but it is not advisable for mothers, who are medically untrained, to do this.
   The temperature of much older children may be taken by placing the thermometer in the child's mouth, under the tongue.
4. Leave the thermometer in position for two or three minutes.
5. Take the thermometer out and read where the end of the silver line is on the scale.
6. Clean again with soap and water.

Fig 14.2
Thermometer being positioned correctly by a qualified nurse.

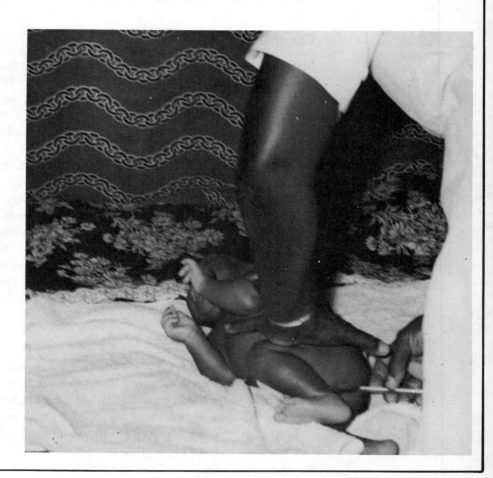

Fig 14.3
Malarial parasites.

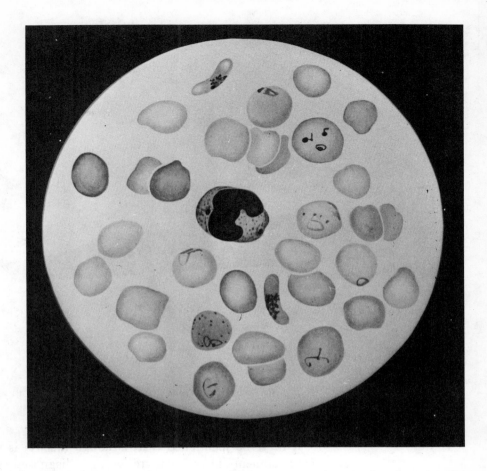

Malaria

This is the most common illness in both children and adults. It is caused by a micro-organism known as a malarial parasite, shown in Fig 14.3. The parasites, which are spread by mosquito bites, feed on human blood and cause anaemia, which is popularly known as 'shortage of blood' (see page 123). The main signs of malaria infection in children are fever, vomiting and abdominal pain.

Malaria is very rare in newborn babies and in infants of less than three months old. This is probably because young infants are still protected by the antibodies they received from their mothers.

As well as causing anaemia, malaria infection may also cause convulsions resulting from the sudden and very high temperature of the malaria fever. Malaria is one of the main causes of failure to thrive in young children. It may also cause the spleen to become large. An enlarged spleen can be felt as a firm swelling at the left side of the abdomen just below the ribs.

The best way to prevent malaria is to eliminate all mosquitoes from the home. If this is not possible, the children should sleep under a mosquito net. Drugs which prevent malaria infection are also available but the disadvantage of using these drugs is that if they are not taken regularly, and the child develops malaria, the infection tends to be very severe.

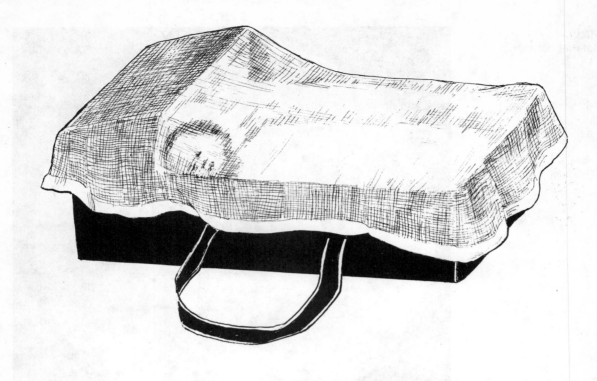

Fig 14.4 Use a mosquito net to protect the sleeping baby.

It must be mentioned that, although malaria is very common, many other ailments in children are wrongly diagnosed as being malaria. The doctor is the best person to diagnose and treat malaria infection.

Diarrhoea and vomiting

Gastro-enteritis is the medical term for diarrhoea and vomiting. It is caused mainly by viruses and is spread in contaminated food or water. Poor hygiene and sanitation are very important factors which are responsible for spreading the infection.

Gastro-enteritis usually starts suddenly. The affected child passes very watery stools which may contain mucus. Vomiting may be mild, moderate or severe or may not occur at all, particularly in newborn babies.

Diarrhoea and vomiting lead to a rapid loss of salt and water from the body. In severe cases, the child may lose weight rapidly. The mouth will become dry, the eyes sunken and the fontanelle depressed. The infant will look weak and dull. Treatment consists mainly of replacing the salt and water, which have been lost, as quickly as possible. The best place for treatment is a hospital or a well-equipped clinic but a mother can help to remedy the loss of water by giving her child water containing sugar and a little salt as frequently as possible.

Boiling all drinking water and observing strict hygiene and good sanitation are the precautions needed to prevent gastro-enteritis in our children.

The common cold	This is also known as 'catarrh and a cough'. It is caused by viruses and is very infectious. Its spread is encouraged by overcrowding and by unhygienic ways of sneezing, nose-blowing and coughing.

Signs of the common cold are the same in all age groups. Sneezing is usually the first sign and is quickly followed by stuffiness of the nostrils which soon begin to discharge watery fluid. Coughing then follows and is often worse at night than during the day.

In young children the common cold should be treated promptly by taking the child to see a doctor as soon as possible. This is because the illness is liable to cause the same complications as in newborn babies, mentioned in Chapter 13. Ear infection is an additional complication which is not found in newborn babies. The ears ache and may discharge pus. Chronic ear infection can cause deafness in children. |
| **Anaemia** | Anaemia is also popularly called 'shortage of blood' although this is not really an accurate description. There are several reasons for children being anaemic. Firstly, their diet may be deficient in protein, iron and vitamins which are all necessary for blood production. Secondly, malaria infection can cause anaemia in children and thirdly, some children have worms in their intestines which cause anaemia as will be explained shortly. Lastly, all infections, especially when they are prolonged, depress the activity of cells in the bone-marrow which are responsible for producing blood.

In children with dark skin, anaemia can be most easily detected by looking at the tongue and gums, both of which look pale. Signs of anaemia can also be detected by looking at the inner side of the lower eyelids, the nails, palms of the hands and soles of the feet. Anaemia can be more easily recognised in light-skinned children.

Eating a good diet and avoiding all infections, especially malaria, are very important in the prevention of anaemia. |
| **Worms** | The worms most commonly found in young children are roundworms and threadworms. A roundworm is a large worm which resembles an earthworm except that it has no rings visible on it. A threadworm, as its name implies, is a tiny thread-like worm. Hookworms which suck blood and cause severe anaemia are fortunately uncommon in young children.

Roundworms and threadworms enter the body in food or drink contaminated with faeces which contains the eggs of the worm. Roundworms deprive the child of whatever food he eats and so cause the child to become malnourished and anaemic. Female threadworms lay their eggs on the skin around the anus causing intense itching. When the child scratches his anus, he picks the eggs up on his fingers and then whatever he touches is immediately contaminated with these eggs.

When a child has abdominal pain worms *may* be the cause but this is often not the case.

Many drugs for deworming children are now available but, as always, a doctor is the best person to advise on which drug to use. It may also be |

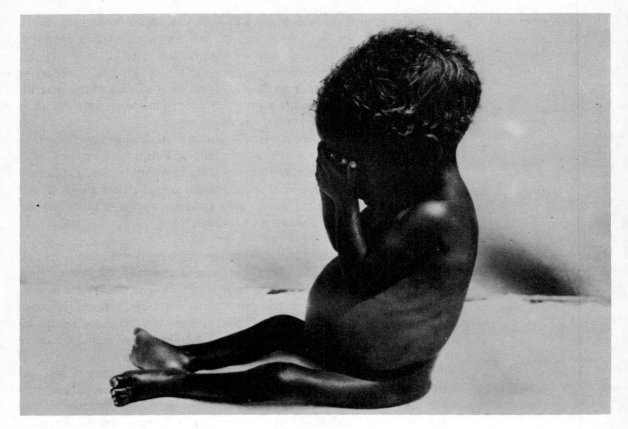

Fig 14.5   A malnourished child.

necessary to examine the child's stool in a laboratory in order to determine which worms the child has.

Malnutrition

Malnutrition simply means bad nutrition or bad feeding. Bad feeding does not only mean inadequate feeding but also includes over-feeding with the wrong foods.

The malnourished child is easily recognisable. He is usually between one year and three years of age. He is small for his age, thin and pale. He has prominent cheeks, flat buttocks and a potbelly. He may have ulcers at the corners of his mouth showing that he is deficient in vitamins. When his malnutrition is advanced, he becomes miserable and refuses to eat. His skin begins to crack and peel and his feet start to swell. The importance of a balanced diet in the prevention of malnutrition was discussed in Chapter 7.

Infectious diseases

All the infections discussed here spread easily from one child to another and can cause epidemics. They are the most common of all the infectious diseases. Fortunately, the first five of these infections can now be prevented through immunisation at the infant welfare clinic (see page 99).

Measles

This dangerous disease is caused by a virus and can be avoided by immunisation (see page 101). The signs of measles are well-known to most experienced mothers. The illness begins with catarrh and a cough accompanied by a redness and soreness of the eyes and mouth. The child's temperature rises steadily and is not lowered by the usual anti-fever drugs. The child is miserable and refuses to eat. After four or five days, the measles rash appears on the face and spreads rapidly to the rest of the body. The rash does not usually itch much.

Heat rash and rashes caused by other infections are often mistaken for the measles rash. The measles rash is recognisable because it is always accompanied by catarrh, a cough and redness of the eyes and mouth.

Complications of measles include pneumonia, diarrhoea and vomiting, convulsions, severe skin and eye infections and malnutrition. These are more likely to develop if the child is not treated promptly. Children still die from measles because proper medical treatment is not begun early enough. Children suffering from measles will easily pass on the disease to other children near them. This is why immunisation is so important. Any children who have been near to an infected child should be taken to see a doctor as soon as possible.

Whooping cough

This infection is caused by bacteria. The illness is recognised by the child's prolonged coughing which ends with a whistling noise known as a 'whoop'. The noise is made when the child takes a deep breath while coughing. The child may vomit at the end of a bout of coughing.

Pneumonia and convulsions are the serious complications arising from whooping cough. There may also be bleeding into the eyes, resulting from the rupture of a small blood vessel during a bout of coughing.

Whooping cough may last for several weeks or months. Even after the child has recovered, he may start to 'whoop' again if he develops a cold. This 'whooping' may recur as long as six to twelve months after an attack of whooping cough but this does not mean that the infection has returned.

Tuberculosis

Tuberculosis is a public health problem in many parts of the world. This is why the BCG vaccine is now given to babies to protect them from tuberculosis (see page 101). The disease is caused by slender and delicate-looking bacteria. Children with tuberculosis have a chronic cough, a fever and will lose weight. The glands in the neck may become enlarged causing a swelling to appear in the neck. The spine may also be affected, developing a lump which may result in the child becoming hunchbacked. Tuberculosis may also affect the abdomen and the brain.

Tuberculosis in children is not very infectious. In other words, a child with tuberculosis does not easily spread his infection to others. It is *adults* who have tuberculosis who are responsible for spreading the infection.

Modern medicine has produced many drugs to combat tuberculosis so that doctors now have several drugs to choose from. Tuberculosis can now be completely cured. However it takes between eighteen months and two years of steady treatment to cure the patient. This is an important fact to note as some parents of affected children stop bringing their children to

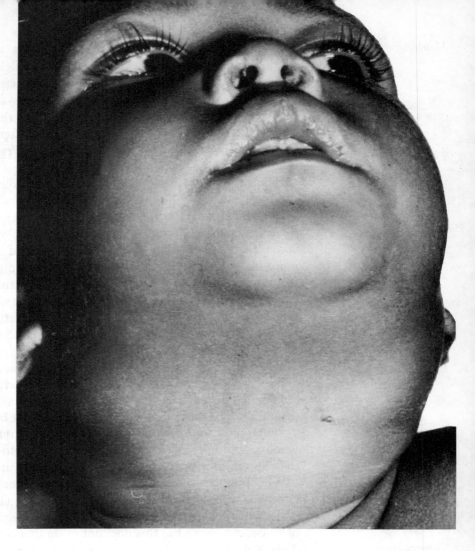

Fig 14.6
Swollen neck glands
caused by tuberculosis.

the hospital before the doctor has finished the necessary treatment. In such cases, the disease often returns in full force after a few months and the doctor must then start the treatment all over again.

Poliomyelitis

Many people who are crippled have been victims of poliomyelitis, often simply called polio. The infection is caused by a virus and affects mainly young children. It starts with a fever, catarrh or a cough and sometimes vomiting and diarrhoea. A few days later some parts of the body, usually one or both legs, become paralysed. Paralysis is very painful and the child will cry whenever the affected area of the body is touched.

Until paralysis appears, it is very difficult to diagnose poliomyelitis. Illnesses such as malaria or the common cold are often wrongly diagnosed when the child really has polio. The child may then be given an injection because his illness has been wrongly diagnosed. When a limb later becomes paralysed, the parents may then wrongly blame the injection, and the doctor who prescribed it, for the paralysis.

Poliomyelitis is also difficult to treat. Treatment consists mainly of resting the patient in bed and relieving the pain with drugs. When the pain subsides the patient may be sent for physiotherapy which consists mainly of special exercises designed to help the muscles to recover.

Babies are now given a polio vaccination to prevent the spread of the disease (see page 101).

Diphtheria

Bacteria are responsible for this dangerous infection which, fortunately, is not common. The infection causes a severe form of sore throat in children. The glands in the neck are swollen and may become very large. The child's neck then resembles that of a bull and he is said to have 'bullneck'.

The occurrence of this disease has been greatly reduced by immunisation (see page 101).

Fig 14.7
A child crippled
with polio.

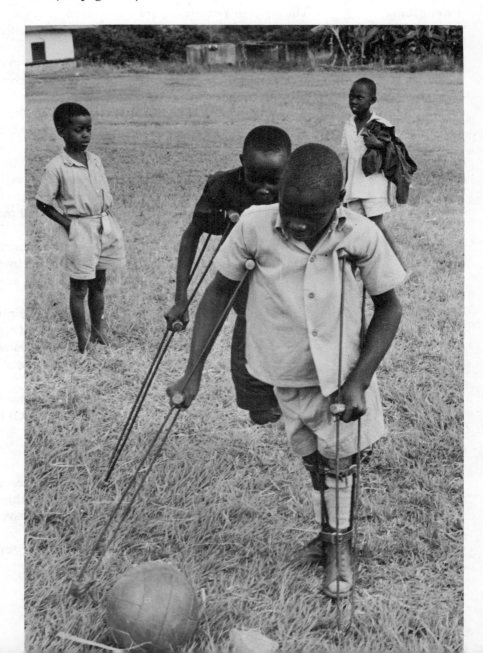

Chicken-pox	Chicken-pox is not common in very young children. It occurs more often in older children and adolescents. Chicken-pox resembles impetigo except that the chicken-pox rash causes considerable itching. Also, the fluid in the chicken-pox rash does not turn to pus.
Mumps	Mumps is also uncommon in very young children. It causes swelling on one or both sides of the jaw. The swelling is painful and takes three weeks or more to subside. A child can only suffer from the illness once; this is because the child's body will automatically become immune to the illness after he has had the first attack. It is important that boys should have mumps before puberty as the illness can cause great pain and sometimes impotence in adolescent boys and men.
Pneumonia	The signs of pneumonia are well-known. They are fever, a cough, chest pain and fast breathing. Young children may develop pneumonia from a common cold which has been neglected.
	Various bacteria and some viruses can cause pneumonia. By carefully examining the child and taking an X-ray of his chest, doctors can usually tell which bacteria is responsible.
	Pneumonia is one of the commonest causes of death in children in hospitals. This is mainly because the children are brought into the hospital too late for treatment.
Dysentery	This is an infection of the bowel. The patient has diarrhoea in which the stool is small, loose rather than watery and contains blood and mucus. The diarrhoea is accompanied by a colicky abdominal pain and straining while passing stools.
	Like gastro-enteritis, dysentery is caused by contamination of food or drink with faeces. Children often get dysentery by picking up and eating dirty food from the floor.
Skin infections	In newborn babies, skin infections are caused mainly by bacteria. In older infants and young children, several other types of organisms can also cause skin infections. There is therefore a greater variety of skin infections which can be caught by children after the newborn period. Some skin infections can arise from insect bites.
	Skin infections often result from poor hygiene. However it should be stressed that some children are more prone to skin infections than others.

Convulsions

Although they are not one of the 'top ten' diseases, convulsions are one of the most frightening illnesses in children. The three main causes of convulsions are high fever, brain disease and epilepsy.

High fever	When convulsions are caused by a high fever, they are described as **febrile convulsions** and are usually found in children aged between five months

and six years. Febrile convulsions are by far the most common type of convulsions in young children and tend to run in families. If one or both parents suffered from febrile convulsions in childhood, the children may inherit the tendency to have febrile convulsions.

The fevers which cause febrile convulsions start suddenly and the temperature of the child rises rapidly. Not all infections cause this type of fever. The infections which most often do this are malaria, the common cold, measles, sore throats and ear infections. Febrile convulsions do not last for more than ten or fifteen minutes. The child should be cooled with tepid water to ease the convulsions. He then recovers except for the signs of the infection which caused the fever and gave rise to the convulsions. He should be taken to a hospital when the convulsions have stopped.

A child who has suffered from febrile convulsions tends to have repeated attacks until he reaches the age of six or seven years when the attacks usually cease. The attacks can be prevented with certain drugs.

Brain disease

Convulsions caused by brain disease are usually prolonged and more severe than febrile convulsions. The child may have two or more attacks in a single day and may not regain full consciousness at the end of the convulsion.

Epilepsy

Epilepsy is a hereditary disease. However, it may skip several generations. It is therefore often difficult to know from which relative the child has inherited his epilepsy. Epilepsy is not infectious. The child is quite healthy apart from his epileptic attacks and with the aid of modern drugs can lead a normal life.

What to do

Death from convulsions is usually the result of wrong handling of the patient by his parents and other relations. If the following rules were always observed there would be fewer deaths from convulsions.
1. Don't panic.
2. Place the child on his side on a flat surface and remove all tight clothing.
3. Try to cool the child down by sponging him gently with cool water.
4. Arrange to take the child to a hospital and take him there as soon as possible. Make sure that he lies as described in (2) while he is being taken to the hospital.
5. Do not touch or handle the child unnecessarily as this merely prolongs the convulsions.
6. Do not put any objects in the child's mouth. He will very rarely bite his tongue.
7. Do not give the child anything to drink. He may choke as he is unconscious and cannot swallow.
8. Do not rub oil or ointment on the child's body. This is useless and only wastes precious time.

When the child arrives at the hospital, the medical staff will do the following.
1. Give the child an injection to stop the convulsions or to prevent further attacks if the child has stopped convulsing.
2. Sponge the child with cold water if his temperature is very high.
3. Examine the child to find out the cause of the convulsions.
4. Carry out other necessary investigations which may include putting a needle into the child's spine.
5. Give the child any other necessary treatment.

Some wrong beliefs about convulsions are still held but should be ignored. The following are some of these beliefs.
1. Modern or 'European' medicines are useless in the treatment of convulsions.
2. Injections can cause convulsions.
3. Giving an injection to a convulsing child can cause death.
4. Convulsions are infectious.
5. If a convulsing child is allowed to clench his teeth he will die.
6. Putting charms on a child or scarifying the face keeps away convulsions.

Glossary

afterbirth	the placenta, delivered after the birth of the baby
ambidextrous	describes a person who can write equally well using either hand
amniotic fluid	fluid surrounding the foetus in the womb
anaemia	popularly called 'shortage of blood'. One cause of anaemia is a shortage of red pigment in the blood, a sign of a deficiency of iron in the diet
antenatal appointment card	a card kept by the mother and shown on each visit to the clinic
antenatal card	a record of visits to the antenatal clinic
antenatal clinic	a clinic for expectant mothers
antibodies	various proteins in the body fluids important for fighting disease
anti-tetanus serum	a drug given to a newborn baby whose mother was not immunised against tetanus during pregnancy
areola	the dark area on breast around nipple
asphyxia of the newborn	a serious condition in infants who fail to breathe immediately after birth
bonding	the close emotional link between mother and baby
brucellosis	a disease causing abortion in women
Caesarian section	an operation to deliver a baby when normal birth is not possible
canine teeth	the teeth on either side of the incisors
colostrum	the rich breast milk produced in first few days after birth
febrile convulsions	convulsions caused by a high fever
foetal-alcohol syndrome	a dangerous condition of the foetus caused by excessive drinking of alcoholic drinks by mother during pregnancy
foetus	the unborn baby
fontanelle	a small depression in the baby's head where skull bones meet
gari	one of the many names for cassava porridge
gastro-enteritis	medical term for diarrhoea and vomiting
genes	substances in every cell of the body at birth which determine the expression of inherited characteristics

hypothermia	a condition caused by a severe reduction in the temperature of the whole body
immunisation	the administration of a vaccine to protect an individual from various diseases and infections
impetigo	a skin infection causing blisters and then ulcers
incisors	the four middle teeth in upper and lower jaws
infant welfare appointment card	a card given to a mother at the clinic with information for her guidance
infant welfare clinic	a clinic for infants of between six weeks and five years old
infant welfare record card	a record of the baby's progress measured on visits to the clinic
jaundice	an illness which causes the skin to have a yellowish colouring
kwashiorkor	a disease in children caused by lack of protein in the diet
leptospirosis	a lung infection
micro-organisms	tiny living creatures visible only through a microscope
midwife	a nurse with extra training in pregnancy and childbirth
modified milk	commercially produced cows' milk which has been modified to resemble breast milk
molars	the two pairs of upper and lower back teeth
neonatal tetanus	a disease spread by infection of the umbilicus in newborn babies
paediatrician	a doctor who specialises in children's health
palpation	the abdominal examination held at the antenatal clinic
pap	a preparation made from maize or sorghum (guinea corn)
penicillin	a type of drug given by a doctor to fight some diseases and infections
perinatal mortality	the proportion of babies who die within the first week of life
perinatal period	the first week of a baby's life
placenta	the source of nourishment to the foetus inside the womb
post-natal clinic	a clinic at the hospital or maternity home for babies of up to six weeks old
primary vaccination	the first vaccination given against smallpox
salmonella	micro-organisms which cause dysentery and food poisoning
septicaemia	blood-poisoning
sphygmomanometer	a machine used to measure blood pressure

syphilis	a venereal disease harmful to the foetus
thalidomide	a tranquillising drug which is now known to cause deformities in the unborn baby
thermometer	an instrument for measuring body temperature
toxaemia of pregnancy	an illness causing high blood pressure in expectant mothers
toxocara canis	a fever spread by a micro-organism in dog faeces
trimester	a three-month period during pregnancy
umbilical cord	the cord joining the foetus to the placenta
vaccination	see immunisation
vaccinia	the smallpox vaccine
weaning	the gradual introduction of an infant to solid foods

Index